Praise for *The Menopause Reset*

Our goal with respect to hormones is to create a healthy physiology so we live a long, loving, active life. Dr. Mindy's book The Menopause Reset *has exactly the right tools to make this happen. She educates on how to do keto, fasting, and diet to enhance hormones and smooth the menopausal transition. This book and her programs are exceptional and are a must-read for every woman who is perimenopausal, in menopause, and postmenopausal.*

— **Anna Cabeca, D.O.**, best-selling author of
The Hormone Fix and *Keto-Green*

• • •

As a doctor and researcher, this book offers some powerful and simple insights into understanding the basic biology of menopause, but more importantly, as a woman starting to forge her own journey into these transformational years, I found The Menopause Reset *to be spot on with what I have learned for myself and thousands of women over decades of practice. Dr. Pelz provides a new hopeful narrative, expectation and outcome for millions of women globally. Dr. Pelz is one of the few colleagues I have met who is all about MASTERING, not medicating, your hormones as you shift from a time of being a care giver to self-care seeker. She reminds us that suffering is NOT normal and that symptoms are simply a call for help. Thank you, Dr. Pelz, for being an empowered voice and leader helping the millions of women already through the doorway of menopause and welcoming those to come. This will be a must read for all of the women in my life.*

— **Dr. Nasha Winters, N.D.**, author of
The Metabolic Approach to Cancer

• • •

Let's be real. The decline in hormones can leave you feeling like you're on an emotional roller coaster. Dr. Mindy lays out some great steps in her book women should follow if they are in perimenopause or menopause!

— **Dr. Carrie Jones**,
head of medical education at Rupa Health

Dr. Mindy Pelz is a pioneer for women's health. Her pain-to-purpose story has inspired many around the world, including myself. The information in this book is unlike anything you've come across before, and it will change your life. What I love most about Dr. Mindy is her commitment to research the root cause of health. Dr. Mindy possesses a rare energy, and a unique gift for breaking down the complex into bite-sized nuggets, which leak out of the pages of this book. I'm blessed to work closely with Dr. Mindy and see firsthand the impact she continues to make in this world.

— **Ben Azadi, FDN-P**, founder of Keto Kamp

• • •

Never have I met a woman so dedicated to empowering and helping the world. Dr. Mindy's passion for health and getting information out to all those in need is prevalent in this book. She is a mentor, a friend, and a force that is going to help shift the health paradigm.

— **Dr. Sonya Jensen, N.D.**, founder of Divine Elements-Naturopathic Family Wellness and co-host of *The Women N Wellness* podcast

• • •

The Menopause Reset *is an extremely relevant book that all women need to read. Dr. Mindy Pelz offers a valuable guide to ditching the symptoms so that you can feel like yourself again. She puts the power back in your hands, which is more important today than ever before.*

— **Dr. Caitlin Czezowski, D.C., CFMP, CACCP**, founder of The Dental Detox and co-host of The Women N Wellness podcast

The Menopause Reset

Also by Dr Mindy Pelz

<u>Books</u>

Fast Like a Girl:
A Woman's Guide to Using the Healing Power of Fasting
to Burn Fat, Boost Energy and Balance Hormones

The Reset Factor:
45 Days to Transforming Your Health
by Repairing Your Gut

The Reset Factor Kitchen:
101 Tasty Recipes to Eat Your Way to Wellness,
Burn Belly Fat and Maximize Your Energy

*Available from Hay House
Please visit:

Hay House UK: www.hayhouse.co.uk
Hay House USA: www.hayhouse.com®
Hay House Australia: www.hayhouse.com.au
Hay House India: www.hayhouse.co.in

The Menopause Reset

Get Rid of Your Symptoms and
Feel Like Your Younger Self Again

DR MINDY PELZ

HAY HOUSE

Carlsbad, California • New York City
London • Sydney • New Delhi

Published in the United Kingdom by:
Hay House UK Ltd, The Sixth Floor, Watson House,
54 Baker Street, London W1U 7BU
Tel: +44 (0)20 3927 7290; Fax: +44 (0)20 3927 7291; www.hayhouse.co.uk

Published in the United States of America by:
Hay House Inc., PO Box 5100, Carlsbad, CA 92018-5100
Tel: (1) 760 431 7695 or (800) 654 5126
Fax: (1) 760 431 6948 or (800) 650 5115; www.hayhouse.com

Published in Australia by:
Hay House Australia Ltd, 18/36 Ralph St, Alexandria NSW 2015
Tel: (61) 2 9669 4299; Fax: (61) 2 9669 4144; www.hayhouse.com.au

Published in India by:
Hay House Publishers India, Muskaan Complex, Plot No.3, B-2,
Vasant Kunj, New Delhi 110 070
Tel: (91) 11 4176 1620; Fax: (91) 11 4176 1630; www.hayhouse.co.in

Text © Dr Mindy Pelz, 2020 and 2023

Indexer: Jay Kreider
Cover design: Julie Davison
Interior design: Bryn Starr Best

A catalogue record for this book is available from the British Library.

Tradepaper ISBN: 978-1-83782-013-9
E-book ISBN: 978-1-4019-7440-4
Audiobook ISBN: 978-1-4019-7441-1

Printed and bound in Great Britain by Clays Ltd, Elcograf S.p.A.

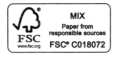

*Dedicated to the three people
who matter to me most in this world:
my husband, Sequoia, and
my kids, Bodhi and Paxton.*

*Thank you for always being in my front
row, cheering me on and loving me
through my menopausal madness.*

I love doing life with you!

Contents

Foreword

To those of you who don't feel well, can't lose weight, and have said, "I have tried everything," let me give you hope. You are not alone, and believe it or not, there is something you haven't done yet to get to the cause of your symptoms.

I have a saying: "If you fix the cell, you will get well." This was true in my life and now it has helped millions of others. The reason you still don't feel well and it's harder to lose weight or even stick with a diet? It's a hormone problem. However, the cause of this problem is, in fact, your cells. I have taught thousands of doctors from around the world this simple concept, and there is a growing group of us resonating with this message. It seems so simple and yet not enough people are asking, much less searching to understand, what it actually means and how to apply it.

In *The Menopause Reset*, you will learn in a clear and simple way how to fix your cells and get your life back. I have been blessed to teach a concept for many years referred to as the Pompa Protocol, which is a multi-therapeutic approach to fixing the cells and, ultimately, your hormone problems. Fasting, feast-famine cycling, diet variation, and cellular detox are all part of this cellular solution you are about to learn.

Dr. Mindy Pelz has taken this life-changing message to so many whom I could have never reached, and for that I am forever grateful. She suffered from the typical perimenopausal and menopausal symptoms that so many women deal with today. Her authority comes from this.

She can speak to it from her perspective and take what I have taught to another level of understanding.

"From pain to purpose" has been my mantra for many years because all I teach has come out of my own battle with an unexplainable illness. I was not a woman struggling with menopause, but I suffered symptoms from the typical to the bizarre. It started like most chronic illnesses do, with fatigue, anxiety, and brain fog. It then progressed to insomnia, being hypersensitive to every food or chemical, and losing the ability to deal with even normal stress. I couldn't even handle loud noise and crying kids. My thyroid was not right—my hair was thinning. I was constipated. I became "skinny-fat," and my energy was gone. My adrenal glands were fried as well. Yet my blood work was still normal. I couldn't even deal with the stress of picking out a shirt for the day. Seriously, it would make me anxious and overwhelmed. I, like most people with these symptoms, tried many treatments for my thyroid, adrenals, and other hormones, but all of it was too far downstream from where the real problem was. How did I, Dr. Mindy, and now millions of others get our lives back? We determined the upstream cause and fixed our cells using these strategies.

I would be remiss if I didn't tell you that out of the thousands of doctors and practitioners I have taught, Dr. Mindy stands in a special class. I call them Three Percenters. Three Percenters change the world. They don't make excuses but plow ahead even in great adversity. They live it to lead it. They innovate. They never stop thinking of ways to bring something that makes a difference in others' lives to more people. Most of all, they are called to something greater than themselves, and they just seem to know it. They rise to what God has called them to do.

Dr. Mindy has done just this in *The Menopause Reset.* If you take this information and put it in practice, your life *will* change. This is what Three Percenters do. They hear the truth, make no excuses, and jump in with all they have. When research was conducted on people who have done extraordinary things like beating cancer or other incurable diseases, the researchers asked them what their secret was. The most common answer? They just made a decision one day. They made a decision to get well or to do whatever it took to get well. They chose. You too can choose to be a Three Percenter and get well. Here is the truth: choose it now!

—**Dr. Daniel D. Pompa**
Author of *The Cellular Healing Diet*
and *Beyond Fasting*
Park City, Utah

CHAPTER 1

Whose Body Am I Living In?

Can we get real for a moment? Menopause is crazy hard. Sleepless nights, erratic moods, weight-loss resistance, memory loss, hot flashes, thinning hair, vaginal dryness, and loss of libido are not a walk in the park. Menopause is not like handling a bad flu that comes and goes in a matter of weeks. It's a decade-long journey during which our bodies shift in massive ways. Symptoms seem to have no rhyme or reason. They come and go with no warning. Hormones that have kept you happy, mentally clear, energized, and burning fat are no longer there. We miss them. But they are not coming back. This hormonal decline is a turbulent, crazy, wild ride we go through alone and aren't given enough solutions to. I want to change that.

Why don't women share their experiences with this menopause journey more often? Why aren't we giving women better lifestyle tools to deal with this? Why aren't women supporting each other through this process? Menopause is an extreme sport. We need a training manual on how to prepare for this adventure. We need to lean into each other and help each other out.

After spending the past 10 years moving through my menopause journey, I now realize I was not alone. Too many women are having similar experiences. Some have it even worse. Women struggle with their health when they hit this time of life. It sucks when your life gets turned upside down as your hormones decline. Thousands of you have reached out to me. Your stories have moved me. So much so it inspired me to write this book.

My 40s were the beginning of a downward spiral for my health. I hit my 40th birthday in the best shape of my life. I was pretty sure aging was going to be piece of cake. Yet, by 42, my health had unraveled. Hot flashes, insomnia, memory loss, erratic moods, and unexplained weight gain became my reality. I felt like I lived in someone else's body, like an alien had taken over my body. I no longer felt in control of my health. The worst part of this journey is that all my old tricks I used to use to get my health back on track didn't work anymore.

One of the toughest parts of the menopausal years is that the symptoms are complex and unpredictable. We often never know when they will come or how long they will last for, and it's hard to pinpoint what initiates them. For years, many of us have learned to come to peace with our PMS symptoms. That was easy in comparison to the transition into menopause. PMS provides us a short, hormonal change that just happens right before our periods. We've found tools to manage them (one of those tools being lots of chocolate). Yet the menopausal hormonal journey is different. It doesn't have the same predictability. Symptoms come and go with no signal, showing up at the worst moments possible.

There are so many emotions that go along with this crazy hormonal roller coaster. Our relationships can suffer because of our erratic moods. Anger and agitation become frequent visitors. For some of us, we find ourselves yelling more at our kids and partners. The smallest situations can easily provoke us. The hardest part is that we often don't know why. We often walk around just feeling irritable.

I've coached thousands of women through their menopausal journey who've told me they've completely lost the joy in life. It's frustrating when the small things that brought you joy in your younger years doesn't provide you the same excitement. Many women find their memory fades during these years. Too many, find themselves in the middle of a conversation searching for words and forgetting names. A restful night's sleep can feel like a luxury of the past for many menopausal women. Any movement or noise easily wakes us. Once awake, we spend hours tossing and turning, trying to get back to sleep. Many nights we wake up drenched in sweat, forcing us to get out of bed to change our clothes and sheets. Too many of us during this time would give anything to wake up feeling rested.

And the weight gain. Can we talk about the weight gain for a moment? It's not fair. Do you feel like you are eating the same (maybe even less), exercising more, and all you seem to do is gain weight? Menopause sneaks up on you. Too many of us feel too young to be going through menopause. Menopause was something that happened to your mother when she got old. That's not you. That can't be the point of life you are in.

As difficult as this journey may be for you, I want you to take a step back from your symptoms for a moment to give yourself a new perspective. Suffering through menopause is optional. Seriously, it is. The symptoms you are experiencing are cries for help from your miraculous body. You don't have to struggle through them. You are way more powerful than that. The menopause journey is a beautiful opportunity to tune in and find out what your body needs.

Everybody needs something different. I want to help you build a lifestyle that is personalized to what your body cries for. Symptoms are gifts. I know they don't feel like that while they are occurring; but if your body had a language, it would talk to you in symptoms. Try not to villainize the process. Tune in and listen to it. These symptoms show up for a reason.

I get how hard it is to live in a body that doesn't feel like yours. I know these symptoms may suck the joy out of your life. You've tried everything to feel better, and nothing feels like it is working. The number of herbs, supplements, medications, therapies, and diets you have implemented to feel normal again is vast. You are out of answers and massively frustrated. I've got you. Help is on the way. Look at this book as an instruction manual on how to smooth out the menopausal ride. Your menopause journey can be an inside-out experience. Instead of looking for something from outside you to cure your symptoms, I want to teach you how to live a life that supports the changes happening inside you—a lifestyle that honors the wisdom that your body has within. Doing so will cause your external experience to change. I want to teach you the language your body is speaking and give you the tools to work with your body and not against it.

You will see that I am a science nut. It's not enough for me to just know that something works; I want to know why it works. I built my whole practice around using healing tools that not only are effective, but also have the research to back up why they work. One of the most startling pieces of information I discovered when going through

my menopause journey was that diseases like breast cancer, ovarian cancer, heart disease, diabetes, dementia, and
Alzheimer's more commonly happen to women in their
postmenopausal years. I wanted to know why that was the
case. What happens that sets women up for so many diseases? What I discovered is that our hormones are like a
symphony. Each instrument plays a part in making a beautiful piece of music. If one of those instruments breaks, the
whole piece will be off. It's in this breakdown of a few hormones that disease sets in. Balancing our hormones as we
move through menopause is not just about keeping our
sanity; it's also about saving our lives.

I am on a mission to help women understand this. If
we course-correct through a woman's menopausal years,
we can help her prevent serious diseases like cancer, heart
disease, dementia, Alzheimer's, and even osteoporosis.

I am honored to be on this journey with you. I am a
true believer that everything in our life happens for a reason. I know my struggles through menopause happened
so I could find answers for thousands of women going
through this process. Keep an open mind as you read this
book. Many of the lifestyle tools I recommend are cutting
edge, but they may be the opposite of what you have been
taught up until now. Science teaches us differently. The
world we live in today is different than it was decades ago.
Because of that, we need to do menopause differently.

I've got great news for you. Wherever you are in your
menopausal journey, you can change these symptoms.
And quickly. It doesn't take a magic pill; it can be as simple
as making changes to your lifestyle that will work with the
hormonal decline you are experiencing. I am excited to
share with you the lifestyle tools that I found have helped
me and thousands of my patients smooth this ride out.

I don't believe in magic pills. I believe in the power of the human body. The design of the female body is incredible. We were built to grow another human being inside of us. How cool is that? But it's this design that shifts dramatically during our menopausal years. You don't need a magic herb or an antidepressant medication to cure that shift. You need a shift in your lifestyle to meet the changes that are happening inside you.

Knowledge is power. The more you understand about what your body is going through, the more in control you will feel. Understanding hormones is complex. This book is designed to simplify them for you so you can work with your hormones and not against them. You can stop your symptoms. You can thrive through menopause. You have more power than you've been taught. I am excited to give you that power back.

CHAPTER 2

●●●●●●●●●●●●●●●●●

Welcome to Menopause

I'm probably the most unlikely person to be writing a book on menopause. For most of my life, I had few struggles with my hormones. My period came and went with few symptoms. I never experienced any challenges with fertility. When I turned 30 and my husband and I decided we wanted to conceive a child, I got pregnant right away. I put little thought into how to balance my hormones. Then I hit my 40s. My hormones took me on a course I never knew I'd experience. It was a wild ride, and it took me a decade to figure out how to get off.

I wrote this book because I felt alone through this process. My symptoms were intense and dramatically affecting my life. Yet the only answers I could find were to suffer through the process or medicate it. I didn't like either of those options.

Since I have been sharing my menopause journey on social media, I have heard from so many of you who have had similar experiences. Menopause has hit you hard, too. Like me, you didn't see it coming. My menopause journey started in my early 40s. Overnight, I went from being a joyful, energetic, and kind person to being an emotional, hot mess. Seriously, I felt like someone hijacked my brain and was in control of my thoughts, sleep, and well-being. It was disruptive to my life and my relationships and left me not loving the person I turned into. It also became the catalyst for a decade-long quest that has allowed me to not only stop my own hormone madness, but also turn around and help thousands of women who are going through the twists and turns of their menopause journeys.

When I turned 40, I had one goal: to be in the best shape of my life. At that point in my life, that meant fitting into my favorite pair of skinny jeans or seeing a certain number on my bathroom scale. I thought that being healthy meant eating well and exercising a lot. My measurement of health was an outside experience. If I liked how I looked on the outside, then I assumed all was well on the inside.

My 40th birthday quickly came and went. I had heard grumblings from other women who'd turned 40 about just how hard it was to lose weight. I didn't experience that. I felt invincible. My life was in a sweet spot. I had two amazing kids who were 10 and 8 at the time, a loving and devoted husband, a thriving wellness practice, and an incredible community of friends.

Within months after my 40th birthday, I began to experience deep waves of depression. It hit out of the blue and had me crying for no specific reason and left me feeling joyless. At first, the waves were small and infrequent, but as my 40s went on, they became more and more frequent. I'm a make-lemonade-from-lemons kind of gal, so it took me some time to clue in and recognize just how depressed I had become. I kept using all my mindset tools to regain my joy, but nothing was working. None of this made sense. There was no trigger, no traumatic event, nothing in my life that I could point my finger at and say, "That's it. That's why I feel so blue."

What I learned from those years of depression is that there will always be moments in our lives that bum us out. Situations don't go the way we plan and leave us depressed. Up until my early 40s, I had experienced that kind of depression. But this felt different. The only way I could describe it is that it was deep and illogical. I wanted to withdraw from my life that, on paper, was the American dream. My heart goes out to those of you who have struggled with this kind of depression before. It's tough. It was like something had taken over my brain and I was no longer in control.

At this point in my professional career, I knew a whole lot about physical health and little about mental health. I went digging for information on tools like diet, exercise, chiropractic, acupuncture, and methods of mindfulness, like meditation and yoga. I read inspiring books, listened to motivational speakers, and leaned on the wisdom of friends who had walked the path of depression before. All these tools helped, but only temporarily.

Waves of depression soon turned to panic attacks. Anxiety became a frequent visitor. I would wake up at night with this deep sense of dread. Many nights, I would do what I called my worry scan. Two in the morning would hit, and I would be awoken out of deep sleep. Panic, fear, and anxiety would take over. My mind wanted to attach a reason to this panic so I could understand it. I would quickly scan all the parts of my life in which something went wrong. For the next two hours, I would toss and turn, trying to solve problems in my mind that in some cases didn't exist. It felt like insanity, but I couldn't make it stop.

Then the nightly hot flashes kicked in. They were so bad that I would have to change my clothes multiple times in one night. My sheets would be so drenched, I would have to wake up my husband to change them. I started sleeping in a sleeping bag in our bed so I didn't have to wake him. Between the anxiety and hot flashes, sleep became a hurdle. It would be easy to say this was the classic beginning of menopause, but I was 43 years old with a regular cycle. The average age for the onset of menopause is 55.

This was true hell. This was not what I expected health in my 40s to look like. I knew something was hormonally wrong with my body; I just couldn't figure out what was causing it. What lifestyle tool was I missing? More importantly, how was I going to pull myself out of this?

In times of crisis, I have never been afraid to reach out and ask for help. Luckily, I had an amazing community of wise women that surrounded me. I started off by reaching out to my big sister. She confirmed that she had experienced some depression and anxiety at my age and found antidepressants to be a good solution. Her recommendation? Maybe it was time to turn to medication. It was tempting. Take a pill and this nightmare would all go away. I hadn't taken any medications in years, and as a holistic doctor, I knew that taking medication was only a patch, not truly addressing the root cause. I also was familiar with studies done on long-term health consequences of chronic antidepressant use. Perhaps the biggest downside of antidepressant use is once you get on them, it's hard to get off. I wasn't willing to mess with my neurochemical system so drastically. I didn't want to rely on a medication to make me happy for the rest of my life. There had to be another solution. There had to be a reason I felt this way.

I reached out to my friend group, many of whom were 5 to 10 years older than me. Their response to me was, "Buck up. You're entering perimenopause. Get ready for the ride; it's a brutal one." At 43 years old? It still didn't make sense. I remember my mom bragging for years how easy menopause was for her. She went through menopause in her early 50s without a hot flash or depressing moment in sight. There was no doubt I was missing something.

One night, I was at my kid's school science fair when I found myself standing next to one of the moms who was a well-respected OB/GYN in our community. I was desperate and out of answers, so I approached her and told her about my situation. Her response to me dramatically changed the way I looked at health forever.

She said, "Mindy, I wish I had an answer for you. I have a practice full of women your age who have those hormonal symptoms, and I honestly don't know what to do with them. My medical textbooks have failed me." That was not the answer I expected. The words "a practice full of women who have those hormonal symptoms" and "my medical textbooks have failed me" rang in my ears for weeks after our conversation. If it was happening to so many women, there had to be an environmental piece to this hormonal puzzle.

That night changed everything for me. It was the catalyst for discovering the tools I used to reset not only my menopause symptoms but also, now, those of thousands of women. These tools took me years of research and persistence to understand and apply, but they are what gave me my life back, and they will do the same for you.

Our conversation that night ignited an insatiable desire inside me to figure out why this was happening to so many women and what I could do to solve my health crisis. It led me down a path of compelling research that is proving we have an epidemic of depression, anxiety, hormonal imbalances, weight-loss resistance, and thyroid problems in women today. And, yes, the medical textbooks have failed us.

For the past decade, I have been deeply invested in understanding the effect today's toxic world has on women. I have also been obsessed with all the research proving to us how powerful our bodies are at detoxing themselves using tools like fasting and the ketogenic diet. I can honestly sit here at 50 years old and tell you I am a happier, healthier, more vibrant version of my 40-year-old self. The tools I lay out for you in this book gave me my joy and sanity back. I easily sleep through the night and wake up rested. Night sweats are a rare visitor. Depression can't find its way into my brain. When the occasional anxiety attack sneaks up on me, I'm prepared and have tools to quickly turn myself around. I feel powerful and in control. I feel like me again.

My menopause journey ignited a burning desire in me to teach women how to do this time of their lives differently. We don't have to suffer. We don't have to build disease. We can use our menopause experience as an opportunity to reset our health and be our best for years to come. I see these protocols work again and again for women. I have become so passionate about the opportunity for menopausal women to reset their health that I rebuilt my clinic around this concept. I built online programs such as the Women's Metabolic Reset and those in my Reset Academy, which bring together women in a supportive community environment and teach them tools they can use to overcome their symptoms. And lastly, I created a detox program that is specifically targeted at removing the toxins that destroy women's hormones.

Don't ever lose faith in yourself. You were born in the most amazing, self-healing body. You just need to learn to tap into that healing process. I'm excited to be on this journey with you. You deserve to live a joy-filled life.

This book is a summary of my findings and the path I used to regain not only my health but also that of the women in my practice and virtual community. It is my gift to you. From the bottom of my heart, I hope you find the answers you have been looking for here.

CHAPTER 3

Reset Your Menopause Symptoms

No matter where you are in your menopause journey, I want to teach you how to reset your symptoms. The next few chapters hold some incredible tools for you to change the direction your health is heading. When I set out to write this book, I was clear that I had one goal in mind: to teach women how to heal themselves from their menopause symptoms. The hero of the day is not your doctor, the quick-fix diet your friends are on, or a magic pill that will take all your symptoms away. The hero is *you*. The magic is within you.

Your body was designed to heal. There is a lifestyle that will maximize that healing. But it isn't as simple as just going for a jog or doing one three-day water fast. You will need to implement several lifestyle changes to thrive during these years. Your toolkit may include intermittent fasting, the ketobiotic diet, eating to feed your hormones, detoxes to rid yourself of toxic estrogens, and mindfulness techniques. Over my years as a holistic doctor, I have observed that when people first decide to try a more alternative, natural way of healing, they bring with them the mindset that is taught by conventional medicine. The one diagnosis, one pill mindset. Think about blood pressure. You walk into your doctor's office and find out your blood pressure is high. What will your doctor do? Most likely give you a diagnosis and prescription, right? Let's say you don't want to take that medication. You want a more natural approach. So, you go hunting for that one thing that will bring down your blood pressure naturally. But what if there isn't one thing that caused your blood pressure to go up? What if there were many causes? One natural supplement won't be your cure.

That's what you will find with your menopause symptoms. There is most likely not one specific issue causing your symptoms. There are, most likely, several causes. Don't be discouraged by this. What I have done is mapped out five major lifestyle changes you can make to feel well again. These include adjusting when you eat, changing what you eat, feeding your microbiome, lowering your toxic load, and balancing your stress levels. We will dive into these five parts of your life in detail. I will show you what the latest research is proving to us about how these habits affect our hormones.

First, I will teach you how your body works. Then I'll give you solutions to work with your body so it performs better. Last, I'll follow this up with steps you can walk through to succeed at the principles. I usually put those steps in order of easiest to hardest. Chapters 4 and 5 are designed to help you understand your hormones during the menopause process. This is critically important, because once you have an understanding of what these hormones do as you move through menopause, you can identify which lifestyle change will most benefit you. Let's go back to the high blood pressure analogy. Imagine if your doctor said, "Here are five reasons why your blood pressure is high," and then gave you five steps you could take to address those reasons. Wouldn't you feel more empowered and in control compared to just being handed a prescription?

Chapters 4 and 5 lay a foundation for the changes you can make to enjoy this menopausal ride. Once you get through those chapters, you will dive into Chapters 6 through 10. These chapters outline the lifestyle changes you can make to thrive through menopause. You may read these chapters and feel like a rock star because you are already doing much of what I present here. If that's you, fabulous. Be sure to read the steps I have laid out at the end of the chapter and ask yourself if you have done all those steps. Most people find there is more they can do to improve their health. If you read these middle chapters and realize you know nothing of what I am presenting here, that's fabulous as well. Go back and reread the chapter. Then follow the steps in the exact order I give them.

At the end of this book, I will show you exactly how to put it all together and give you resources to support you on your menopause reset journey. Whatever you do, don't give up. I purposely put those steps there for you. It's easy when you are overwhelmed with new information for limiting beliefs to show up. You might find your mind saying nonsense to you like, "This is way too hard," or "I could never do this," or "What will my friends and family think of me?" Don't listen to those thoughts. I teach in alignment with how your body wants you to take care of it. You will see that when you work with your body's design, lifestyle changes will feel effortless. I see this all the time. Someone will tell me they have an insatiable sweet tooth and nothing will ever change that; then we fix their gut microbiome, and their sweet tooth goes away. All we did was work with the body's design and the symptom changed.

Here are the five lifestyle changes that make up your menopause reset.

Step 1: Change *When* You Eat

Step 2: Address What You Are Eating

Step 3: Repair Your Microbiome

Step 4: Detox Yourself and Your Life

Step 5: Stop the Rushing

Each step can build on the next. Just like walking a long staircase, take it one step at a time. Before you know it, you will have all the steps put together in a beautiful lifestyle that works for you.

That's what happened for Cathy. At 49 years old, she was at the height of her menopause symptoms. Night sweats, anxiety, memory loss, hair loss, chronic fatigue, rising cholesterol levels, and unexplained weight gain became her new normal. As a high-achieving athlete, she was used to exercising her way out of any symptom. For the first time in her life, exercise was not the cure. In fact, the more she exercised, the worse her symptoms got. When I first started working with Cathy, she was a six-meals-per-day, carbohydrate-loading kind of gal. She had been trained in the "breakfast is the most important meal of the day" mentality.

The Menopause Reset lifestyle was extremely new to Cathy. In fact, many of the tools I recommended to her seemed counterintuitive to what she had been taught about health her whole life. But her old tricks didn't work.

She knew it was time for a change. She dove in, working the steps I outlined above. I started by moving Cathy's breakfast back an hour. At first this was challenging for her. She quickly got the hang of it, though, and within weeks, she intermittently fasted every day. With this first step alone, she felt more energy. The next task I had was to move Cathy away from a high-carbohydrate diet. She started by removing the refined carbohydrates like breads and pastas. This slowed down her hunger, allowing her to fast longer. As she fasted longer, she dropped the belly fat that had accumulated in the past few years.

With her energy up, hunger down, and weight falling off her, I tested her gut to see what type of good bacteria she had working for her. Turned out she was massively deficient in helpful bacteria that bring down cholesterol levels, break down toxic estrogen, and speed up metabolism. She started to add to her diet more plant diversity and polyphenol, probiotic, and prebiotic foods. With this step I saw her cholesterol come down and even noticed changes to her skin and hair.

The last step was to lower her toxic load. Cathy's heavy metal test showed she was extremely high in lead and mercury. I taught her how to remove those toxins safely and effectively, opening up her detox pathways first and then removing toxins from her body and brain. This last step gave Cathy her life back. She started to sleep through the night, the anxiety went away, her hair stopped falling out, and night sweats became a thing of the past.

Although not officially through menopause, Cathy now had the tools in place to keep her symptoms at a minimum. With all the previous steps in place, Cathy looked at her overscheduled life. She built in downtime, said no to more invitations that might drain her, and we even got her to add more variation to her exercise schedule.

Each step was a new way of life for Cathy. Each step felt unfamiliar at first. But as she hung in there, each step got easier and more familiar. The best part is that each step brought back a new level of health for her. I recently ran a hormone test on Cathy, and her hormones looked amazing and well balanced. She was perfectly poised to move through menopause with minimal symptoms and no room for disease.

You can do exactly what Cathy did. She didn't have any superpower that you are not equipped with. Follow the steps. Tap into one of my online programs if you need more support and community. Know that this process works, and it works every time.

As extra fun, outside of the lifestyle changes you can make to smooth your menopause ride, I have also included some cutting-edge tools that will speed up your healing process. Again, this is a lifestyle book. If you love what I have to say in Chapter 11 about staying forever young, be sure you are still working the lifestyle principles of the menopause reset.

You've got this. I have watched thousands of women go through the process of resetting their health. It doesn't matter where you are in your menopause journey: whether pre, mid, or post, you can reset your health. I can't wait to show you how.

CHAPTER 4

●●●●●●●●●●●●●●●●●●●●●●●

You're Not Losing Your Mind— You're Losing Hormones

Menopause could quite possibly be the wildest hormonal time of your life. I promise you that you are not crazy. One discovery I made was how little I truly understood about my hormones. I didn't realize the massive impact they had on my life. I looked at menopause like a switch that got turned on when you reached a certain age. One day you have your period; the next day, you don't. Nothing could be further from the truth. For many women, menopause can be a 10- to 15-year journey in which their ovaries shut down and other organs pick up the hormonal slack. These organs may already be overworked and not up for the job.

I want you to master your hormones. This means having a basic understanding of which hormones have the greatest impact on you throughout your menopause journey. This also means getting to know the organs in your body that produce these hormones. These organs make up your endocrine system. In this chapter, I will introduce you to the endocrine organs that influence your symptoms the most. I will also talk about my favorite strategies to understand your hormonal profile and which hormones you need to work on the most.

Let's go back to how your body is designed. Whether you like it or not, as a woman, much of your design is geared for growing and birthing a baby. From the moment you went into puberty, your body and mind have been under the neurochemical influence of hormones that have a powerful effect on how you feel. If I detailed all the chemicals that surge through you in a 28-day period, you would be shocked at how many neurochemicals have to work together every month to bring you joy, help you sleep, calm you, beautify you, keep your hair full and your skin wrinkle free, lubricate your mucous membranes, ramp up your sex drive, allow you to multitask, motivate you to work out, and even give you the gift of gab. Since you started puberty, you have had a beautiful symphony of hormones that helped you in so many ways. The struggle for the menopausal woman is that all those helpful hormones are now gone.

Your 40s are the beginning of this hormonal decline; but your hormones don't decline in a slow, consistent way. They go haywire. Some days they are higher than normal, while other days they are nonexistent. This is what puts you on that emotional roller coaster and makes you feel like you are going crazy. Essentially, you can have the hormones of a teenager one day and the next day be completely depleted of hormones like a postmenopausal woman.

The highs and lows of my emotions were so intense that I never knew if I was going to be filled with joy and gratitude or if I would want to kill anyone who looked at me wrong. My mental state didn't seem to come from circumstances being right; it felt like something else was in charge, like an alien took over my brain and left me feeling out of control and unpredictable. I hated it, yet it was this crazy up and down that empowered me to get to know my body at a deeper level.

When you dive into understanding hormones, you will see that there are a lot of societal misunderstandings about how the female hormonal system works. For example, did you know that your hormones aren't controlled by just one organ in your body? They are controlled by a team of organs. This misunderstanding is seen a lot with thyroid conditions. When a woman's metabolism goes awry, it's common for her to go see her doctor, who will test her thyroid to see if that organ is working correctly. But that organ doesn't work alone. It has to get directions from the hypothalamus and the pituitary gland in her brain. Treating the thyroid as an isolated organ will never completely resolve a thyroid condition. You need to address the whole team.

Endocrine glands are the organs that produce your hormones. Every endocrine organ works with this team approach. These teams even have their own name. For example, one of the team names you might be familiar with is the HPA axis. This is your adrenal team, which includes your hypothalamus and pituitary gland and the endocrine glands known as your adrenal glands. This team produces cortisol so that you have energy and mental clarity during times of stress. The other team that has been working so hard for you is your sex hormone team called the HPO axis. This team is also made up of your hypothalamus and pituitary, with the endocrine gland being your ovaries. Your HPO axis team controls all production of estrogen, progesterone, and testosterone.

When you enter into your 40s, the HPO axis team begins to slow down. It's done its job for thirty-some years, and it's not interested in working anymore. But your body still needs some sex hormones, so the HPO axis has to hand its duty over to another team. That team is the HPA axis. It's in this handoff where the menopausal madness begins.

For many of you, your HPA axis team has been working overtime for years due to all the physical, emotional, and chemical stress you've been under. When your HPO axis team checks out and hands their job over to the HPA axis team, your sex hormones will decline quickly. This decline will leave you anxious, depressed, unable to sleep, lacking sex drive, losing muscle, gaining weight, and feeling like you are going crazy. This is exactly what happened to me.

The hard part is identifying which team member is struggling and needs help. Because there are so many players in the hormonal game, chasing your declining hormones with herbs or medications will often leave you frustrated and out of answers. If you are willing to roll up your sleeves and dive into understanding your body and all that is involved in your hormonal picture, you can take your health to a higher level than you ever experienced before.

This transition through menopause is critical. So many imbalances in your body will reveal themselves. Understanding these imbalances and committing to fixing them can be life saving. Menopause is an incredible time to reset your health. Our younger years are so much about raising families, building careers, and caring for those around us. The menopause years are an opportunity for us to care for ourselves. We should want to take insane care of our health to be our best in our later years.

Fixing your hormones during these years can feel like a daunting task. At times, taking a pill to resolve your problems can appear attractive. I promise you that if you hang in there and listen to your body, you will not only help your symptoms today, but your tomorrow self will thank you as well. Here's the advice I give women as we put their hormonal picture back together: be patient and build yourself a toolbox.

This is not like repairing a sprained ankle. Balancing hormones is way more complicated than that. As you move through these years, there will still be highs and lows. There is no way around that. But you do have control over how low the lows go. Everyone's toolbox will look different. For example, for many of you, detoxing heavy metals from your hypothalamus and pituitary will balance your melatonin levels and get you sleeping again, while some of you need to lower your carbohydrate levels and learn how to create a fasting lifestyle to kick yourself out of insulin resistance.

Since menopause is a journey, knowing which tool can balance which hormone becomes incredibly helpful. It puts you back in the driver's seat.

Be Willing to Make Yourself a Priority

I know you've been putting all your heart and soul into everyone around you, but now is the time to put your heart and soul into you. Declining hormones mean declining protection. You are more vulnerable to disease during your menopausal transition than ever before. On the pages of this book are some of the greatest tools for resetting your hormones, but nothing will save your life more than you making yourself a priority.

Like no other time in your life, the menopause years will reveal where your imbalances are. If you have been living an overscheduled, stressful life, it will catch up to you. If you have been able to eat whatever you want and not feel ill effects, that may dramatically change as your hormones decline. If you want to thrive during these years, your lifestyle may need a dramatic makeover. But it all starts with taking a deep breath and making *you* the priority now.

This is exactly what happened to Debbie. At 45, not only did she have a high-powered, high-demands job, but she would also come home at the end of the day to the job of taking care of her family. This left little room for her to think about herself. In her early 40s the demands of her life left her little time to focus on herself. She looked at self-care as a luxury, not a key to balancing her hormones. When her menopause symptoms got out of control and she found it difficult to keep up with the life she had created, she came to me for a consultation. I ran a hormone test and found that her adrenals, along with her progesterone, testosterone, and DHEA levels, were tanked. There was no diet or detox that was going to save Debbie until she made herself a priority.

The first step to Debbie's menopause reset was to slow her schedule down. She had to learn to say no and prioritize downtime. Once she made herself the priority, thinking of her hormonal needs first, her symptoms started to calm down.

Don't Guess—Test

Because there are so many players involved in your hormonal picture, this is the time that testing becomes crucial. The test I find the most helpful is a called a DUTCH Complete™ hormone test. The reason I love this test is that it is easy to use and gives us a complete picture of all the hormones at play in a menopausal women's journey.

The DUTCH test is an at-home urine test. You can order this test on my practice's website. The test is performed by taking five different urine samples in a 12-hour period. The results will tell you exactly what is happening with your sex hormones: estrogen, progesterone, and testosterone. It also gives you a reading on how well your adrenals are functioning. This is really helpful when you want to know if your adrenals are producing enough cortisol and at the right time of the day.

It can give you a better understanding of your neurotransmitters like serotonin and dopamine, which keep you happy. This powerful test will also tell you if your body is getting rid of toxins efficiently, or how well you are methylating, which I will go into more detail on below and in Chapter 9. You can even see if your pineal gland is making enough melatonin. Can you see why I love this test? It's so complete and thorough.

Perhaps what I love most about the DUTCH test is its breakdown of your estrogen metabolites. *Metabolite* is a fancy term used to explain what happens to a chemical after it has been broken down, or metabolized. In this case, an estrogen metabolite is an important measurement of what your total estrogen gets broken down into. Sometimes hormones get metabolized into byproducts that are disease forming. This is particularly true with estrogen. If a woman knew what her estrogen was being broken down into, she could prevent many hormonal cancers.

You have three types of estrogen metabolites. One is protective and will help prevent hormonal cancers and cardiovascular disease. Two are harmful and will cause many cancers. Knowing your balance of these estrogens is crucial for not only feeling well today but also preventing disease in the future. Once you know your estrogen metabolite balance, there are detox strategies that you can implement to raise the protective estrogen and lower the harmful estrogen.

I recently had a 48-year-old patient, Megan, run a DUTCH test, and her bad estrogens were incredibly high while her protective estrogens were extremely low. She was also not methylating properly. *Methylation* is just a fancy word used for a cell's ability to detox. Not methylating well can be a problem for a menopausal woman because those toxins will stay inside the cell and cause long-term damage. When I looked at her test, I thought, "Wow, the information here is going to save Megan's life." She was on a fast track to building a hormonal disease such as breast cancer.

It turned out Megan loved to eat out a lot, often without concern for the quality of food she ate. She was a frequent visitor to fast-food restaurants. When I sat with her to read her DUTCH test, I was clear—the time to change her food habits was now. If she didn't clean up her diet, she was on a fast path to breast cancer. That is how powerful the findings of this test can be.

What I love about Megan is she is an all-in kind of woman. When she saw her DUTCH test, it mobilized her. Not only did she change her eating habits, but she also joined my Women's Metabolic Reset and learned how to eat and fast to drop weight. She is now down 40 pounds and feeling better than ever. The best part is we did a comparison DUTCH test and can see her good estrogens rising and her harmful estrogens declining—literally life saving information.

I believe so strongly in the information this test can give you that I recommend every woman, pre- or post-menopause, have one. We could end so much suffering if women better understood their hormonal profiles and course-corrected before it was too late.

I want to make sure you get the most out of this book. I am not looking to give you pieces of information that entertain you; I want this book to change your life. As you move through the following chapters, think about how you can build a hormonal toolbox. The tools I will lay out for you can be taken as steps. Master one step, then move on to the next. I am excited to take you on this journey. You live in such an incredible, self-healing body that wants to work with you, not against you. Don't ever lose faith in yourself. Don't let anyone tell you that you just have to live with your symptoms. You are more powerful than that.

As you move through the next few chapters, keep in mind the principles I have taught you here. Think about Megan, who got tested and decided to make herself a priority and change some of her deadly habits. She course-corrected so that the back half of her life was not built around managing disease. Like no other time in your life, understanding your hormones, making yourself a priority, and building yourself a toolbox can be lifesaving.

Now let's dive in and understand each hormone so you can build the best toolbox for you.

CHAPTER 5

••••••••••••••••••••

Dear Progesterone, I'm Sorry I Took You for Granted

I'm going to be honest with you. Before my menopause journey, I never thought much about my hormones. I never gave them credit for the joy they gave me and how impactful they were on my health. I remember when the waves of anxiety hit me, I dove into understanding progesterone. I never realized that this glorious hormone showed up for me every month to calm me and put my body at ease. Then she disappeared—and I would love to have her back. One anxiety-ridden day, I drove to work and the thought went through my head, "Did I ever take progesterone for granted! What a gift that hormone was for me." I've since learned that many women have no idea which hormone is coming or going and how each contributes to their well-being. Because menopause is the time your sex hormones are surging and declining, it is helpful to understand what these hormones do.

I tell my clients all the time that if they want to balance their hormones and feel like themselves again, they will want to have a basic understanding of the hormones involved in their menopause journey. This is exactly what I did when my hormones spun out of control. I went back to my textbooks and took a deep dive into female physiology 101. Knowledge is power, and I felt powerless. Over the next few pages, I want to give you that power back, too.

The first step to regaining a sense of control is to understand which hormones affect which symptoms. When you have a basic understanding of your hormones, you will know which tools to use.

Let's start with your hormonal hierarchy. Did you know that all hormones were not created equal? Certain hormones have more power over others. This is a key concept that Dr. Anna Cabeca champions in her book *The Hormone Fix*. When you think of menopause, most likely you think of three sex hormones as the troublemakers: estrogen, progesterone, and testosterone. It would appear to make sense that as these hormones decline, you would want to elevate their levels. But there are three other hormones that have a powerful effect on your sex hormones. If you don't balance these three hormones, you will work against your sex hormone decline and never feel like yourself again.

Now, here's the fun part. Guess what hormone is at the top of the hierarchy? Oxytocin. Remember this hormone? If you are a mother, this is the hormone that came surging through you when you held your child for the first time. Remember how incredible that felt? Ever fallen in love? Well, guess what—oxytocin gave you that incredible, yummy feeling inside you every time you saw your loved one. Any animal lovers out there? Guess what makes us feel so calm and relaxed when we snuggle with our pets? Oxytocin.

Oxytocin is the best hormone around. The beautiful part of our hormonal design is that it's at the top of the hormone food chain. When you get lots of oxytocin surging through you, you take a major step forward in balancing your sex hormones. How awesome is that?

The next hormone in line is cortisol. I know, I know. The dreaded cortisol. This is the one that takes your health off course every time. Cortisol gives you the belly fat you hate, makes your blood sugar spike, and will wake you up at two in the morning to tell you there is a crisis going on. Every time you are under stress or perceive you are under stress, your body gives you a good dose of cortisol. Cortisol will even show up when you are overscheduled with fun activities. Cortisol is the hormone of the rushing woman.

This hormone has such a powerful effect on your sex hormones, that I decided to dedicate a whole chapter to help you balance it. I have worked with thousands of women going through the menopausal transition—lowering your cortisol surges is key. You will struggle to lose weight, get a good night's sleep, or feel relaxed in your skin if you don't get your cortisol under control.

Underneath cortisol sits insulin. This is your weight-loss hormone. Insulin is released from your pancreas when you eat. The more sugar in your meal, the more insulin that gets released. If you keep eating a high-sugar, high-carb diet, you will keep releasing insulin. If your body can't handle all the insulin you release into your system through diet, it will store it in fat. That fat can sit there for years until you force your body to go access it. Dr. Jason Fung, author of *The Obesity Code*, was one of the first doctors to bring to our attention that gaining weight was not a calorie-in, calorie-out situation. It was a hormonal one. If you struggle to lose weight during menopause, you will need to have solutions to encourage your body to find the glucose and insulin it stored years ago in fat. It won't be enough to just start changing your diet. This is why I have all my patients going through menopause adopt a fasting lifestyle. I will outline what that looks like in detail in the following chapters.

Now we finally get to your sex hormones. They are at the bottom of the hierarchy, because they can be dramatically influenced by the hormones above. You have three sex hormones that affect you the most: estrogen, progesterone, and testosterone.

Let's start with estrogen. I think estrogen gets a bad rap. In our younger years, you might have blamed your erratic premenstrual moods on estrogen. Our society villainizes estrogen for our emotional sensitivity or the cause of diseases like breast cancers. But estrogen is not all bad. It does help us in many ways.

For most of your life, estrogen has surged in your body around day 12 of your cycle. It's this surge that signals your ovaries to release an egg ready for implantation. If you have kids, estrogen played a big part in ensuring you had an egg ready to go. Without the proper amount of estrogen, you couldn't get pregnant.

Estrogen beautifies you as well. Let's go back to your brilliant design. When estrogen surges and an egg gets released, your body is ready to create a baby. To ensure that you mate, estrogen will make you as attractive as possible. This means thickening your hair; giving you smooth, plump skin; and even adding some extra fat to your hips so that you look ready for childbearing. Yep, believe it or not, there is a waist-to-hip ratio that supposedly makes us more attractive. Estrogen also plays a part in ensuring your vaginal membranes are well lubricated—again, all for procreation.

Now having said all of that, there is a dark side to estrogen that you should be aware of. I mentioned before that we have three types (metabolites) of estrogens: one protective and two destructive. If you allow the destructive ones to build and don't nourish the protective ones, you put yourself in jeopardy of developing hormonal cancers like breast and ovarian cancer. In Chapter 7, I will show you how to eat to build good estrogens, and in Chapter 9, we'll talk about how to not accumulate the bad ones.

The next sex hormone that has been your friend all these years is progesterone. If your hormones were a Disney movie, estrogen might be the evil stepsisters who got all the attention, and progesterone is Cinderella, who had to do all the work with no credit. I didn't fully appreciate this incredible sex hormone until it started to disappear. As I moved into my menopause years, progesterone plummeted and left me with spotty cycles, anxiety, and an inability to relax in my skin.

Progesterone has shown up in your life in spades on day 21 of your cycle. It's what made your uterus shed and bleed every month. Progesterone calms you. It also keeps estrogen from acting up. Estrogen and progesterone have an inverse relationship. If progesterone goes low, estrogen can get out of control. This estrogen/progesterone balance is key to keeping a whole host of menopause symptoms at bay.

Low progesterone often causes challenges for women going through menopause. You know you have low progesterone when you start spotting days before your period. Or maybe you've experienced extremely heavy periods where you feel like you are hemorrhaging. Progesterone often goes low in women during menopause because of the stress demands they went through in their 30s and 40s.

For many women, progesterone goes low as they move through menopause because a steroid hormone called DHEA goes low. Through a series of chemical reactions, DHEA will make progesterone, testosterone, and cortisol. Since your body will always prioritize stress over anything else, if you have spent many years in a stressed-out state, your DHEA stores may have been siphoned off to make cortisol. This can leave you low in both progesterone and testosterone. This is where a comprehensive hormone test like the DUTCH test comes in handy and can tell you your exact DHEA levels. Raising your DHEA levels can help you make more progesterone.

Finally, there is testosterone. You might think of testosterone as a male hormone, but it's an incredibly helpful hormone for women as well. Testosterone helps you in three major areas: sex, motivation, and building muscle. Testosterone is what gives you your sex drive. It is also what motivates you to go after your dreams or to have the drive to work out. When testosterone is high in your body, you will also retain muscle easier as you age. Low testosterone can be a huge contributor to your menopause symptoms. A classic set of symptoms I see with menopausal women is low sex drive, lack of desire to work out, and noticeable muscle loss. That's a testosterone issue.

Now that you understand the main hormones at play in your menopausal journey, here is how this hormonal hierarchy works. When your stress goes up, cortisol goes up. As cortisol rises, so does your blood sugar. When your blood sugar goes up, insulin will rise. This is the point where your body starts storing fat faster than normal. The high levels of cortisol and insulin start to accelerate the decline of your sex hormones, leaving you with insomnia, hair loss, anxiety, hot flashes, brain fog, weight-loss resistance, low sex drive, vaginal dryness, and muscle loss. Sound familiar?

This exact scenario is what happened to one of my patients, Kimberly. She came to me with early menopause symptoms of muscle fatigue, loss of libido, insomnia, unexplained weight gain, and anxiety. At 40 years old, she had lost her groove. She couldn't relax in her skin. She always felt like there was a crisis around the corner. Her stress levels were extremely high. She worked long hours at a demanding Silicon Valley high-tech company. When she wasn't working, she raised two kids. She was the epitome of a rushing woman.

One day, when Kimberly felt like her health was slipping away from her, a friend told her about intermittent fasting.

Being an engineer, she wanted to know exactly how to fast and why it worked. She found my fasting videos on YouTube and decided to apply intermittent fasting to her everyday life. Within a few weeks, she dropped weight. Her energy stopped crashing in the afternoons. She was so encouraged by her results that she decided to take the next step and work on what she ate. That's when Kimberly found my 28-Day Hormone Reset protocol. (In Chapter 7, I will teach you this protocol.) These two major changes brought balance back to her insulin levels. Her health slowly returned, but nothing seemed to improve her muscle fatigue, libido, and anxiety. That's when she reached out to me. I ran a DUTCH test and found that her stress levels had been so high for so long that her adrenals were massively depleted. Her cortisol levels were all mixed up, and her DHEA and testosterone levels were incredibly low. This explained the lingering symptoms.

Let's look at what happened to Kimberly within the structure of the hormonal hierarchy. She started by managing insulin. Bringing balance back to her insulin levels wasn't enough to fix her low testosterone. She needed to rebalance her cortisol levels. That's exactly what we did together. Once I supported her adrenals, brought her DHEA levels back up, and regulated her cortisol levels, she started to feel like herself again. Her anxiety went away, her muscle power came back, and her libido returned. The cool part about Kimberly's story is with her libido back she was now getting more oxytocin. With more oxytocin in the picture, she could help keep the cortisol levels balanced. Keeping the cortisol balanced, she would find fasting much easier. This will allow her to keep those insulin levels down. With oxytocin surging, cortisol well balanced, and insulin levels down, now she can keep her testosterone levels high. See how they all fit together? It's like a puzzle: once you figure out how to solve it, your menopause symptoms will feel more manageable.

We all have a different hormonal picture. It's important to keep in mind that just regulating insulin may not solve all your menopausal symptoms. As I walk you through the next few chapters, keep in mind this is like putting your personal hormone puzzle together.

Now, let's roll up our sleeves and balance your hormones.

CHAPTER 6

●●●●●●●●●●●●●●●●●●

Is Breakfast the Most Dangerous Meal of the Day?

Remember how you were taught breakfast was the most important meal of the day? And that the more you ate, the faster your metabolism would be? Well, I am here to tell you that there is no science behind these two food myths. Believe it or not, breakfast being the most important meal of the day was an advertising slogan that Kellogg's came up with to promote their new cereal, Corn Flakes, back in the 1970s. And eating small meals six to eight times a day has never proven to speed up anyone's metabolism. The key to weight loss all depends on one hormone: insulin.

Balancing insulin is imperative to maintain good health. Believe it or not, this hormone can be the easiest to balance. You have control over your insulin levels every time you eat and when you fast. Resetting your insulin levels becomes a pretty simple task when you start to understand *when* and *what* to eat. In this chapter, I will show you how to best balance your insulin by changing the timing of when you eat.

To better understand how insulin works in your body, let's go back to how your primitive ancestors lived. Even though today we live in a modern world where we've made great technological strides, your body's design has stayed basically the same as it was back in the cavewoman days. In those primitive days, cavewomen didn't have constant access to food. They didn't have refrigeration. In the winter months, they would often go days without access to food. Your body comes preprogrammed to thrive without food. Most of the time, the cavewoman would wake up to no food and have to wait for food to be hunted or collected before she ate. Without morning access to food, her blood sugar would drop. As her blood sugar dropped, her insulin levels dropped. But this didn't hinder her. She was built with an alternative fuel source called ketones. When her blood sugar and insulin levels were low enough, her liver would start making ketones. Ketones went to her brain and made her more alert, gave her energy, and lowered inflammation in her joints. This was all for one purpose: so she could go find food.

Fast-forward to today's world. We don't have to go hunt for our food. We've been taught breakfast is the most important meal of the day. We have been told that the more you eat, the faster your metabolism becomes. Nothing could be further from the truth. You have that same design the cavewoman did millennia ago. You were designed for what we call feast/famine cycling just like your cavewomen ancestors. For many women, going against this design has caused their bodies to secrete insulin all day long. Each time you put food in your mouth, you signal to your pancreas to make insulin. Eating all day long is the fast path to insulin resistance. Your pancreas keeps producing insulin, and your cells eventually can't keep up with the amount of insulin sent their way and become resistant.

The first step in regulating your insulin levels is to change how often you eat. This is easier than you might think. When I sit with a patient for the first time, I work on the timing of her meals before we do anything else. I want to move her from eating all day long with non-stop insulin surges to feast/famine cycling. This is more in alignment with how her body was designed.

If you are new to feast/famine cycling, here is the mindset I want you to have. In a 24-hour period, you should have a window of time when you fast and a window of time when you eat. Up until now, you may have only fasted when you slept. That might be your only six- to eight-hour period without food. This is not long enough to let your insulin levels come down. It's not long enough to reverse insulin resistance or to get your body to secrete ketones. I want you to work toward what is called *intermittent fasting*. The first style of intermittent fasting I want you to master is going 13 to 15 hours without food. Sound like a daunting task? Let me give you an easy way to get there.

The easiest first step toward intermittent fasting is to just push your breakfast back an hour. For many women I work with, this first step can be challenging. You may feel dizzy, hungry, and a little cranky when you first make this change. But remember: you trained your body to expect breakfast. This training has been working against your body's design. Going against your primitive design can have a major influence on how you feel, how much fat you store, and how many sex hormones you make. When you treat your body the way it was designed, you will see how quickly your body will heal.

Once you have mastered pushing breakfast back an hour, now I want you to push it back two hours. Sit with that for a few weeks until that feels easier. As each step of fasting gets easier, keep pushing back your meals until you feel comfortable going without food every day for 15 hours.

Recently, the *New England Journal of Medicine* reviewed the research on intermittent fasting and determined that this style of fasting was incredibly healing to the body. Adopting a life of intermittent fasting can:

- Slow down your aging process
- Improve your memory
- Reverse insulin resistance
- Help you lose weight
- Protect you from neurodegenerative diseases like Alzheimer's and dementia
- Prevent cancers
- Reduce arthritis
- Reverse asthmatic conditions
- Slow the progression of autoimmune conditions
- Increase your lifespan

Intermittent fasting can be a game-changer for you as you move through menopause. This is why I want you to start here before you even look at what food you eat. More on that in the following chapters.

Once you have adopted a life of intermittent fasting, learning how to build a fasting lifestyle can get really fun. If you follow me on social media at all, you know that I teach seven different styles of fasting. Each fast has a different impact on your health. The seven fasts I teach are intermittent fasting, dinner-to-dinner fasting, 36-hour fasting, autophagy fasting, fast-mimicking diet, dry fasting, and three- to five-day water fasting.

Intermittent Fasting

This is what I explained above. The goal is to get you to move toward feast/famine cycling. This is 13 to 15 hours without food. Ultimately, you want to make this type of fasting a way of life.

Intermittent fasting was made popular by a researcher named Dr. Yoshinuri Ohsumi. In 2015, he won the Nobel Prize in medicine and physiology for a discovery called autophagy. In the absence of food, your cells will regenerate. As your blood sugar goes down, it signals autophagy and your cellular intelligence kicks in. Think of autophagy as your cells' way of self-detoxing. Your cells go into a massive repair phase, fixing dysfunctional components inside the cell.

The other hormonal change that happens with intermittent fasting is the production of growth hormone. Growth hormone slows down the aging process and helps you burn fat. It's an amazing hormone. The bummer is that your body is designed to stop making growth hormone around age 30. This is when your body is done growing and will start the slow process of aging. Research is once again proving that the miracles of intermittent fasting will force your body to make growth hormone. You can increase your growth hormone production by as much as 1,300 percent with intermittent fasting alone.[1]

Intermittent fasting is a godsend for menopausal women. This is why I want you to start here. So many of you will see immediate results in weight loss, energy, and mental clarity with intermittent fasting alone. Think about Kimberly's story.

Her first step to balancing her hormones was to control insulin with intermittent fasting. That one step had a massive impact on her health. Once she took that first step and saw some progress, it motivated her to take another step. That's how powerful these tools can be.

Dinner-to-Dinner Fasting

Once you are comfortable with intermittent fasting, I want you to work toward 24-hour fasting. Many people refer to this style of fasting as one meal a day, or OMAD. There are several benefits to dinner-to-dinner fasting. Perhaps my favorite benefit is that it is an incredible way to repair your gut. Research from MIT proved that 24 hours without food triggers your body to make intestinal stem cells.[2] These stem cells will repair damage to the mucosal lining of your gut. This is pivotal for anyone dealing with a gut condition. As you will learn in Chapter 8, you have a whole set of bacteria that break down estrogen. Dinner-to-dinner fasting can help change the terrain of your gut and allow these bacteria to flourish.

Twenty-four-hour fasts also keep your insulin levels low for a longer period of time, forcing your body to go find the sugar and insulin it stored years ago. Many people find this type of fasting so easy and beneficial that they only eat one meal a day every day. I don't recommend you do this fast every day. I recommend that my patients do this type of fasting one to three times a week depending on how deep of a healing response they are looking to stimulate.

Thirty-Six-Hour Fasting

This is the fast you will want to lean into to over-come insulin resistance. I recommend 36-hour fasts to my patients once they are comfortable with intermittent and dinner-to-dinner fasts and want deeper weight loss. The longer you go without food, the more your body has to go find the food it stored years ago. With my patients who are severely weight-loss resistant, I will recommend this fast one time a week until they see the weight dropping.

Seems hard to believe? I have a free fasting group on Facebook called the Resetter Collaborative, and we do a fasting training week once per month. This is an amazing group of people from all over the world who support each other through the fasting experience. I call them my Reset-ters because they are so motivated to reset their health. Every month I teach a different style of fasting. Many times my Resetters will do longer fasts, such as 36-hour fasts, during this week. Over and over again the Resetters who do this training week with us every month see the weight start falling off.

Autophagy Fasting

This is probably my favorite fast for two reasons. First, it gets people great results. Second, it's fairly easy to do. Remember Dr. Ohsumi and his autophagy discovery? Well it turns out that there is an autophagy sweet spot. It hap-pens somewhere between 17 to 72 hours. When you fast in this range your cells go into massive repair. This is fabu-lous for slowing down the aging process, reducing inflam-mation in joints, and stimulating weight loss.

There are two requirements to stimulate autophagy. One is to fast a minimum of 17 hours (you can go more if you want). The other is to keep your protein intake to under 20 grams for the entire day. When you combine these two principles, you stimulate autophagy and your body will repair itself.

Fast-Mimicking Diet

This type of fasting was made popular by Dr. Valter Longo, a researcher from University of Southern California.[3] He discovered that when you keep your calorie intake somewhere between 800 and 1,000, avoid animal protein, and keep protein under 20 grams, you can stimulate stem cells.

His research was done on both type I and type II diabetics. He found when he put them through five consecutive days of these requirements for three months in a row, the body made enough stem cells to repair injured pancreatic cells. How cool is that? When his research first came out, it was difficult to understand what food and fasting requirements he used in his studies. Luckily, he now makes the foods he used available to the public. The program is called ProLon®. I recommend ProLon to my patients who want the benefits of a longer fast but don't want to do longer three-to-five-day fasts. Prolon is very helpful for people like Cathy, who struggled with fasting. She couldn't go longer than 13 hours without feeling dizzy. I tried all my fasting tricks: upped her good fat the day before, lowered her carbohydrate intake, and worked with her to help her slowly push her breakfast back an hour. Nothing helped, so I put her on ProLon for five days. That was the trick. It was the gateway into a fasting lifestyle. After her five-day experience with ProLon, she could easily move into longer fasts like autophagy fasts and 36-hour fasting.

Dry Fasting

There are a lot of urban myths about dry fasting. Let me clarify here what it is and what it isn't. Dry fasting is when you go 12 to 24 hours without food or water. The only research we have to date on this style of fasting is what has been done on the Muslim community when practicing Ramadan. There are several key healing effects of dry fasting. The first is it signals to your body to make brain-derived neurotrophic factor (BDNF). This is like fertilizer for the brain.

It can help you grow new neurons in your brain that help with memory and learning.

The other effect dry fasting can have is that it lowers inflammation. This can be helpful for the menopausal woman who is struggling with arthritis or chronic pain issues.[4]

The third benefit of dry fasting is it can help balance cholesterol. Research has proven that dry fasting can increase your HDLs (good cholesterol) and decrease your LDLs (bad cholesterol).[5] The last benefit of dry fasting to the menopausal woman is that it can help prevent osteoporosis. Your body will secrete a hormone called parathyroid hormone (PTH) during an intermittent dry fast. PTH helps with bone reabsorption and bone formation and increases calcium levels in your blood.[6]

As wonderful as the benefits of dry fasting sound, I want to give you a few words of caution. First off, I don't recommend you dry fast longer than 24 hours. Your body was not designed to go days without water. Second, many people feel that dry fasting for one day gives you the same effect as water fasting for three days. I have searched high and low for that research and can't find it. Dry fasting is not a replacement for longer water fasts. Having said that, I do see my patients often get into a deeper ketosis when they dry fast for 24 hours compared to water fasting for the same time period.

Many of my patients love the fasting so much they play with the different fasts to see which one gives them the best result. Some are a little nervous to dry fast. But Karen, a postmenopausal woman who was concerned about osteoporosis, wanted a fast that could help her best with bone density. She read the research I posted on my website about dry fasting stimulating parathyroid production and was motivated to give it a try. She took my recommendation and only did 12 hours to start. Every week she implemented one 12-hour dry fast. After several weeks, she became comfortable with dry fasting and decided to extend it to 24 hours. After three months of weekly dry fasting, she noticed that she was dropping weight quicker, had better mental clarity, and when she went back to her doctor for a bone density scan, her bone density had improved. The miracle of fasting.

Three- to Five-Day Water Fasting

This is the queen of all fasts. As intimidating as it sounds to go three days or longer without food and only drinking water, it can be a miraculous experience. Dr. Valter Longo was the one who made this fast popular in recent years. He discovered patients with cancer who went through chemotherapy could reboot their whole immune system if they went three days without food. Old immune cells like white blood cells, T helper cells, and CD4 cells that were ineffective and worn out would regenerate after three or more days on a water fast. This regeneration process happened from the secretion of stem cells. I recommend this fast to patients who want to prevent cancer, repair injured body parts, or are looking for a deeper cellular reset. A three- to five-day water fast a couple times a year can be miraculous to slow the aging process, unstick your metabolism, reboot your immune system, and regenerate injured brain cells.

How do you decide when to use all these fasts? This is why I call it a fasting lifestyle. Ultimately, I want you to be comfortable knowing how to use all seven types of fasts. I know that some of these fasts can seem overwhelming, especially if you are new to fasting. But the research is clear: fasting heals. As you go through menopause, you need that extra healing. Menopause is a pivotal time. If you learn how to cycle these fasts, you can dramatically slow the aging process.

Most of my patients cycle their fasts on a weekly basis. I recommend they start with a 5-1-1 variation. Five days a week they intermittent fast 13 to 15 hours. One day a week they do a longer fast, working toward 24-hour dinner-to-dinner fasting. And one day a week they don't fast. This is a great place to start with building a fasting lifestyle. Other variations I have encouraged patients to do are 4-2-1 or 3-3-1 variations.

The 4-2-1 variation is for people who want to drop more weight. Four days a week you fast 13 to 15 hours. Two days a week you extend your fast to dinner-to-dinner fasting. One day a week you don't fast. Again, this is a useful variation if you want more weight loss.

Lastly, I use a 3-3-1 variation for patients who are in a severe healing crisis or are massively weight-loss resistant. This variation has a lot of fasting in it. Three days a week I have them do autophagy fasting, three days a week they do dinner-to-dinner fasting, and one day a week they extend their fast out to 36 hours (I know that is a bit longer than a week). As far as the longer fasts, like three- to five-day fasts, I recommend two times a year for keeping yourself optimally healthy and disease free.

Be playful and curious with these fasts. If you want to understand how these fasts work and which one is best for you, join my Resetter Collaborative. It's a free group on Facebook: http://bit.ly/Resetters. It's a great place to get your feet wet with fasting. I have many new fasters in the Resetters, and you will meet people in that group from all over the world who have had incredible results with fasting. Take Theresa, for example, a 47-year-old Resetter who likes to vary intermittent fasting, dinner-to-dinner fasting, and three-day water fasts. She has been doing that for the past year and has dropped 47 pounds. How cool is that?

When Shouldn't You Fast?

Now that I have gotten you all excited about fasting, let's talk about when not to fast. This is crucial for you if you are in the middle of your menopause journey. If you still have a cycle, I strongly recommend that you don't do a longer fast the week before your cycle. This is a time you need to make progesterone. If you fast for 24 hours or longer, you can cause your progesterone levels to drop even lower than they currently may be. Intermittent fasting is okay during this time. A common question I get is, "What if I don't know when my cycle is coming?" I recommend that if you have a cycle, start tracking it, even if it's all over the place, and be sure you don't go into longer fasts (24 hours or longer) if you are past day 21 of your cycle. If you still get a cycle but it's sporadic, a helpful tool I have found is the Clue app. It's an app you download on your phone and enter the day your cycle starts. It is a simple way to track your ever-changing cycle. Once you have gone a year or longer without a period, you no longer need to follow the above advice. You can fast whenever. My final advice to you on building a fasting lifestyle is to not get overwhelmed. If you are reading through these fasts and having trouble imagining yourself doing the longer ones, start small. Fasting can be fun once you get the hang of it. When you take food out of the equation, miracles can happen.

RESHMA'S STORY

At 49 years old, Reshma started her fasting journey with intermittent fasting for 16 hours every day. She found numerous benefits with intermittent fasting, like more energy and some weight loss here and there. For many years, she had been battling SIBO, a gut dysbiosis that caused severe abdominal pain and bloating. She had great success in managing SIBO with diet but wanted to try adding in fasting. As soon as she added intermittent fasting to the diet that worked for her, she lost a ton of weight. For the first time in years, she was encouraged that she would feel healthy again.

Like many of us do, once Reshma started to feel healthy again, she let loose on her food habits and intermittent fasting. Weight gain and gut symptoms crept back in. She knew she had to get back on track. That's when I customized a fasting lifestyle for her. At first, she was hesitant to fast longer than intermittent fasting. But she had read about so many people having incredible results with fasting that she wanted to give it a try. I had her start by extending her fasts to 18 hours twice per week, and adding a dinner-to-dinner fast once per week. She eventually fell so in love with these longer fasts that she even swapped a day out for dry fasting.

With this new fasting regime in place, weight dropped off her. It was so exciting. But her bloating still persisted. I encouraged her to throw in some longer fasts, like 48 hours. This made all the difference. She lost even more weight, and the bloating went away.

Just as she was finding her fasting groove, she developed a new symptom of pain in her left ear. It persisted. She went for a hearing test and CT scan, but all was normal. In the back of her mind, she wondered if it was tied to her gut issues. She had had such success with fasting, that she decided to see whether her ear symptoms would disappear if she upped her fasting game.

One morning, she woke up and said, "That's it. I'm fasting for seventy-two hours." By the third day of this longer fast, the pain just disappeared. It was like a miracle. She was convinced: fasting heals.

Fasting for 72 hours has now become a ritual for her to heal anything that ails her. The amount of energy she has during her fasts is incredible. Her brain fog disappears. She even gets more creative. She is a recipe creator, and her creativity in the kitchen is amazing when she fasts. She rarely experiences the bloating she had when her SIBO condition would flare up. Pain disappears when she's in a 72-hour fast. The best result of all is that she is 15 pounds away from her goal weight. When she started her fasting journey she was 171 pounds. Today, she is down to 135 pounds. Fasting is truly miraculous.

Next Steps to Building a Fasting Lifestyle

- Move breakfast back an hour.
- Keep moving breakfast back until you are comfortable going 15 hours.
- Make intermittent fasting (13 to 15 hours without food) a normal daily routine.
- One day a week, do a dinner-to-dinner fast.
- Once you have mastered the above steps, you are ready to start experimenting with the other fasts.
- Join my Resetters group and try our Fast Training Week to exercise your fasting muscle.

Fasting can heal your body in so many miraculous ways. If you are new to fasting and feel unsure, I highly recommend you work on the above steps. I have seen the most timid of fasters get the hang of fasting quickly. Fasting heals. I'm excited for you to experience it firsthand. Now let's talk about what the heck you should eat once you open up that eating window.

CHAPTER 7

Ketogenic Solutions for Menopause

Now that you understand the principles around when to eat, let's talk about *what* to eat. In this chapter, I want to teach you which foods help raise those declining hormones. If you are like many women, you have spent much of your life chasing calories. When you wanted to lose weight, you ate less and exercised more. We call this the "calorie-in, calorie-out" strategy to weight loss, and it's one of the worst ways to go about losing weight. Just look at the obesity epidemic we have. So many women are starving themselves by eating only chemical-laden, low-fat foods and trying to burn off those foods with long hours at the gym. Not only is this approach to weight loss hard to sustain, but it also messes with your metabolism and makes it harder to lose weight in the future. I'm not telling you to stop exercising; I'm telling you to stop counting calories.

If you don't count calories, what do you count? Remember, this book focuses on helping you use your lifestyle to balance your hormones. Your calorie intake will not necessarily improve the roller-coaster ride your hormones are on. Controlling the types of foods you eat will.

From this point forward I want you to think of your food in terms of macros. *Macros* is a term we use for the macronutrients that make up the calorie content of your food. The three macros I want you to focus on are carbohydrates, protein, and fat. Each of these macros will serve a different purpose in your menopause journey. Each will raise your insulin levels differently as well.

Remember the hormone hierarchy? Insulin influences sex hormones. If you want to begin the process of balancing estrogen, progesterone, and testosterone, you first want to make sure the types of food you are eating aren't constantly spiking your insulin levels.

A good place to start in understanding how your diet affects your insulin levels is to look at the yearly blood work your doctor runs for you. When you go for your yearly checkup with your doctor, she will normally do a complete blood analysis. In this blood test, there is a measurement called hemoglobin A1C. Hemoglobin A1C tells you what the trend of your insulin levels have been for the past three months. You want that number under five for disease prevention and under three for longevity.

The second way to understand how much insulin your body might be producing is to monitor your blood sugar levels closely with a home blood sugar reader, which you can easily find at your local drugstore. When your blood sugar levels go up, insulin will go up. This is the best way to measure your blood sugar levels regularly. There are lots of good at-home monitors out there, but the one I recommend to our patients is the Keto-Mojo. I encourage all my patients to take a morning blood sugar reading. You want that reading to be between 70 and 90 milligrams per deciliters (mg/dls) on most days. If it is consistently higher than that, you may be forcing your pancreas to make too much insulin, throwing off your whole hormonal cascade.

How do you keep your blood sugar and insulin levels down with diet? It all comes back to your macros. Let's break down each one of these macros so you can better understand them.

Carbohydrates

Of the three macronutrients, carbohydrates will typically raise your blood sugar and insulin the most. Refined carbohydrates, such as breads, pastas, and sugary treats, will have the strongest impact on insulin. Fibrous carbohydrates like fruits and vegetables will spike your blood sugar less and therefore cause less of an insulin surge.

One of the first steps in controlling high insulin amounts is to remove refined carbohydrates from your diet. Just like intermittent fasting, this one change alone can dramatically improve your menopause symptoms. If you combine intermittent fasting with a no-refined-carbohydrate diet, you may immediately see your energy go up, hunger drop, and mental clarity improve. I see this happen all the time with my patients. Once you have accomplished this step, your next step is to start counting your macros. I recommend when you first learn the principle of counting macros that you track your macros with an app. There are many good apps out there to help you do this. The one I prefer is called Carb Manager.

Start entering your food into the Carb Manager app every day. To keep your blood sugar and insulin in a healthy zone, you want to keep your net carbs under 50 grams. Notice that I said *net* carbs. Don't worry, the Carb Manager app will calculate the net carbs for you. But it is important to know that there is a difference between total carbs and net carbs. Net carbs are your total carbohydrate load minus the fiber. Fiber is great for breaking down harmful estrogens—I want you to have lots of fiber.

When you keep your net carbohydrates under 50, your blood sugar should drop into the healthy range of 70 to 90. When you drop into this range, it should signal to your body to make ketones. Ketones are a sign that your liver has made the switch from burning carbohydrates for energy to burning fat for energy. This is a beautiful thing. When you train your body to make that switch, you will find weight loss will come more quickly.

Ketones are also massively healing to your brain, especially the hypothalamus and pituitary, the parts of the brain that coordinate all hormone production. On your blood sugar reader there is a setting for ketones. You want to see your ketone reading above 0.5. We call that nutritional ketosis and the range we are looking for is somewhere between 0.5 and 5.0. As long as you are in that range, you are burning fat for energy. Before I move on to protein, I want to point out an important part of lowering your carbohydrate load. Once you see how well your body works in this low-carb state, it will be tempting to keep lowering your carbs. This often means sacrificing vegetables. For the menopausal woman, this is a bad idea. You need vegetables to break down estrogen. You will see in chapters to come that I have a whole strategy for you to feed the bacteria in your gut that breaks down estrogen. I am not a fan of low-keto diets for menopausal women. Low-keto diets often involve keeping carbohydrates under 20 grams. Instead, I advocate a ketobiotic diet. Ketobiotic means you keep your net carbs around 50 grams, allowing for plenty of greens and probiotic- and prebiotic-rich foods to break down estrogen. I will dive into more detail on probiotic-rich foods in Chapter 8.

Protein

When it comes to protein, there are two things I want you to think about. First is the quality of the protein. Of all the foods you eat, meat can be the most toxic. The animals we eat are often injected with antibiotics and growth hormones, and they are usually fed a high-grain diet. Whatever they put into that meat goes into you. These chemicals can wreak havoc with your hormones. The first step when it comes to your protein is to eat clean. What that means is whenever possible, you want to choose grass-fed, organic meats. I call this clean meat. Start reading labels and looking at what is going into your meat. You will start to see that many meat labels read "Raised without antibiotics," "Grass-fed," or "Hormone-free." After you have committed to eating clean proteins, let's look at the amount of protein you eat. It's common that when someone goes low carb, they increase their protein load. This is not a worthy exchange because protein can raise your insulin levels as well. It is best to keep your protein intake to under 50 grams a day. If you are using Carb Manager to measure your net carbs, just be sure to plug in your protein, too. When you first are trying to understand what your macro loads are, this way of measuring can come in really handy.

Fat

The third macro I want you to start measuring is fat. Just like protein, we have good and bad fat. Eating the good and avoiding the bad is crucial as you move through menopause. Here's why. You are made up of trillions of cells. On the outside of those cells are receptor sites that receive hormones and allow them to move into the cells for activation. Once a hormone is able to get into the cell and do its job, you will feel good. These receptor sites are easily blocked by two things: toxins and bad fats. A blocked receptor site is the kiss of death for a woman going through menopause. Remember, you are already making fewer hormones than ever before, so if the hormones you are making can't move into the cell because of a blocked receptor site, your menopause symptoms will be exacerbated. This is why the first step to monitoring your fat macro is to be sure you are eating good fats, not bad ones.

The most common good fats are:

- Olive oil
- Avocado oil
- Coconut oil
- Grass-fed butter
- Raw nuts and nut butters
- Ghee

Fats you want to avoid are:

- Canola oil
- Vegetable oil
- Partially hydrogenated oils
- Soybean oil
- Margarines
- Corn oil
- Safflower oil
- Sunflower oil

Another important concept to remember is that you want fats to be organic and not rancid. Those hormone receptor sites can get clogged with pesticides. Nonorganic fats are packed with pesticides. When you commit to only organic fats, you skip the dose of pesticides. Fats can also go rancid if they are old. Rancid fats will inflame the cell membrane and make it hard for hormones to get in as well. In my household, we buy smaller bottles of oils and replace them more frequently so that they don't turn rancid on us. You can tell pretty easily if your oils are rancid by smelling them. There is a distinct wet cardboard smell to an oil that has turned bad.

Once you have cleaned up your fats, the next step is to look at how much fat you eat. Go back to your Carb Manager. You want to make sure that over 60 percent of all the food you consume in a day comes from fat. I don't recommend you count grams when it comes to fat, count percentages.

One key nutritional principle to always keep in mind when it comes to eating fats is to be sure to always eat healthy fats. Good fat not only nourishes your cells but also heals your brain, slows down hunger, and gives you nice, consistent energy all day long. I know for many of you it's scary to think of eating that much fat, but I promise you the key to balancing your hormones and losing weight is in lowering your carbohydrate load, moderating your protein, and increasing your fat. I have seen this work over and over again for thousands of women.

If the previous information is new to you, I want you to start by getting comfortable with these diet changes before you do anything else with your food. Many of you will stay in the aforementioned three steps (lower carbs, moderate protein, increased fat) for months before moving on to the next steps. When I work one on one with a patient, I make sure that they are following these steps for at least 80 percent of their week. Once they have a routine of eating this way, then we move on to the next step: eating for your cycle.

Eat for Your Cycle

What I am about to teach you should have been taught to you when you first hit puberty. I don't know why we don't teach all women that they have different nutritional needs at different times of their cycle. You have all kinds of hormones surging at different times of the month, and you can support these hormones by eating certain foods at specific times in your cycle.

I realize that many of you either don't have a cycle or your cycle is irregular, so it would be tempting to skip this step. Don't. Let me teach you the principle of eating for your cycle first and then let's talk about how you map that out for where you are on your menopause journey.

While you were ovulating, you had two phases of ovulation: the follicular phase and the luteal phase. The follicular phase is from day one to 14 of your cycle. This is the phase when your body is preparing to release an egg for ovulation. The second phase you go through in a month is called the luteal phase. It occurs from days 15 to 28, and it is when your uterine lining gets ready for a fertilized egg to implant. At this point in your life, the most important thing for you to understand about these two phases is that there are two times in a 28-day period when you get a massive hormone surge: days 12 to 14 and days 21 to 28. The first surge is when your body needs the best estrogen, and the second is when it needs the most progesterone.

As you move through your menopause years, estrogen and progesterone are rapidly declining. This decline is what is making your periods erratic. It's also what is contributing to your symptoms. Once you recognize this, you can eat certain foods at certain times of the month to support the production of both estrogen and progesterone.

Now hang in there with me. I know this gets tricky, but I'm going to simplify it for you. The first thing to know is which foods increase estrogen and progesterone. Here are some of my favorites.

Estrogen-building foods:

- Flax seeds
- Sesame seeds
- Soybeans/edamame
- Garlic
- Dried apricots, dates, prunes
- Peaches
- Berries
- Cruciferous foods like broccoli, cauliflower, and brussels sprouts

Progesterone-building foods:

- Beans
- Potatoes
- Squashes
- Quinoa
- Tropical fruits
- Citrus fruits

At first glance, you will notice that many of these foods are higher in carbohydrates. You might even be asking yourself, "How can I keep my carbohydrate load under fifty grams and eat potatoes and tropical fruits?" This is where eating for your cycle comes in. Here are the three circumstances I see most often among my patients as they move through menopause. Most likely, you will fit into one of these three categories.

You Still Have a Regular Cycle

If you still have a regular or semiregular cycle, I want you to track it. I like to use the Clue app. Here I am at 50 years old tracking my cycle more consistently than I did as a teenager. I laugh at myself now. But eating for my cycle has been so helpful in mitigating my menopause symptoms that I have become diligent about recording my cycle (when it comes) and eating to build hormones.

Once you are in the routine of tracking your cycle, I want you to pay attention to the two hormone surges discussed above. During the estrogen surge, which typically happens on days 12 to 14, I recommend that you don't count macros and eat as many estrogen-building foods as possible. During the progesterone surge, which typically happens around day 21 and continues until you bleed, I want you to eat as many progesterone-building foods as you want. The same rules apply as in your estrogen-building days: you are not counting macros. I call this style of eating a 28-Day Hormone Reset, because it will have an effect on insulin, estrogen, and progesterone.

I have taught so many women this trick to regulate hormones, and almost every time, I get the questions "Won't I gain weight?" and "Won't that throw me out of ketosis?" Usually, this comes from women who have had great success following the first steps I laid out in this chapter and become fearful to make too many lifestyle changes because they feel so good.

If these are your concerns as well, here's what I want you to do. On these hormone-surging days, you can still intermittent fast. Make sure you fast at least 15 hours during this time. When you are not in a hormone-surge time of the month, I want you to be disciplined about keeping with the macros I set at the beginning of this chapter and lean into some longer fasts like autophagy fasting or dinner-to-dinner fasting. For weight loss, throw in some 36-hour fasts anytime between days 1 and 12 and again between days 15 to 21. This variation will allow you to build hormones when your body needs it and still get the benefits of ketosis when your body is not trying to make these key hormones.

Still not convinced? Let me tell you that I speak from personal experience. When I first discovered how great I felt with a low-keto and fasting lifestyle, I would rarely eat carbs and did long fasts often. This tanked my sex hormones and sent my menopause symptoms into a frenzy. My progesterone was so low that my cycle started getting sporadic. I went from spotting with my cycle to hemorrhaging so bad I thought I needed to stay home from work to manage my blood flow. I was anxious and extremely irritable the week leading up to my cycle. The anxiety would get so bad, I couldn't even relax while sitting at home on the couch. These are all signs of extremely low progesterone. Once I committed to the 28-Day Hormone Reset protocol I mapped out here, the madness stopped. Literally, everything from spotting and hemorrhaging to the anxiety completely calmed down. I now can feel my cycles slowing down as I move through menopause. But it's a gentler and calmer ride. I'm off the roller coaster, and it feels more like my ovaries are slowly shutting down. It's not like the wild ups and downs I had a few years back.

You Have an Erratic Cycle

What do you do if you are not sure when your cycle is coming? This is common the closer you are to the post-menopausal phase of your life.

My first piece of advice is when your cycle does come, track it immediately. Even if you bleed for one day. Make that day one of your cycle. Then follow the 28-Day Hormone Reset. For many of my patients who have erratic cycles through their menopause experience, the 28-Day Hormone Reset can bring back some regularity to their cycles. Remember that the average age to get to the other side of menopause is somewhere between 52 and 55. If you enter into menopause before 50, it can be a sign of an imbalance in your body that needs to be addressed. Following the above strategy often fixes these imbalances and makes your cycles regular again. Now, what do you do if you get to day 28 and you still have no sign of your period coming? If this is you, I want you to pretend that day 29 is your day one, even though you don't have your period. Go back to your Clue app and mark it as day one. Then follow the 28-Day Hormone Reset starting from the beginning. If your period doesn't show up, continue this 28-Day Hormone Reset until you are officially postmenopausal. If your period does show up at some point during this reset, just start at day one of the 28-Day Hormone Reset from the moment you see blood. Keep doing this routine until you are postmenopausal.

You Have No Cycle

What do you do if you are postmenopausal or you are not sure where you are in your menopausal journey but haven't had a period in years? If you are under 50, I want you to follow the 28-Day Hormone Reset as I mapped out above for the woman with an erratic cycle. Remember, there is a good chance you went into menopause too early. For many of the women in my practice who have lost their cycle before 50, following the 28-Day Hormone Reset will have them starting their periods again. This is because you are balancing insulin and your sex hormones with this style of eating.

If you are over 50 and haven't had a period in over a year, you are most likely officially postmenopausal. For you, the hormone-building days are not as crucial because your ovaries are no longer active. But you still need some estrogen and progesterone. You will find that some hormone-building days can be helpful. You also will thrive on a more ketobiotic diet and can usually do longer fasts whenever you want. You don't need to think about timing, but you do need to still focus on hormones. What I recommend is that 80 percent of time you are ketobiotic, using the macros I laid out at the beginning of this chapter (50 grams net carbs, 50 grams protein, greater than 60 percent fat) and 20 percent of the time you eat to build hormones (not counting macros). In a week's schedule, you would spend one or two days hormone-building and the rest week on a ketobiotic diet.

Confused? I know for some of you this is a new approach to food. I summarized it for you below. Be sure to follow the steps in the order I laid out. If you move on to eating for your cycle before you have mastered the keto-biotic approach, it will be difficult. Master ketobiotic first, then try eating for your cycle. If you are not sure when your cycle is coming or going, just follow the 28-Day Hormone Reset. You can't go wrong eating that way because you will still be lowering insulin with the ketobiotic approach and building good estrogen and progesterone with hormone-building days. Just in case you are still lost, I have summarized that 28-Day Hormone Reset for you at the end of this chapter as well.

REBECCA'S STORY

Rebecca is a 59-year-old postmenopausal woman I have been working with for several years. She has a busy life filled with lots of social events, work, and travel. When I first started working with Rebecca, one of the challenges she had was just keeping consistent with fasting and keto life—not because of a lack of desire, but because her schedule was so full she found it hard to get some momentum. I wanted to find a solution for Rebecca that let her get the results she wanted but give her the flexibility to still have fun with friends.

What worked amazingly for Rebecca was one of the resets I created for my community. The 15-day Women's Metabolic Reset varies the different fasts and eating styles to specifically help women lose weight. Being able to do this reset several times a year was key for Rebecca. Over the last year, she has done this reset several times and lost 25 pounds. It has been an amazing solution that allows flexibility with her social calendar, while still giving her the weight-loss results she desires. She finds that whenever life derails her or she feels out of control, she just leans into the 15-day Metabolic Reset. It is easy to follow and has the variety she needs to get back on track.

Weight loss is not the only positive result Rebecca has had. When she jumps on the 15-Day Reset, she gets more energy, her inflammation goes down, her muscle stiffness improves, and her mood is lifted. I love that she has this tool to help her.

Next Steps to Eating to Balance Hormones

- Remove refined carbohydrates.
- Keep your carbohydrate load under 50g net carbs.
- Eat clean protein.
- Keep protein intake under 50 grams.
- Eat good fat; avoid bad fat.
- Be sure that over 60 percent of the food you eat in a day comes from healthy fats.
- Once these steps are mastered, move to the 28-Day Hormone Reset.

In the past few years, the ketogenic diet has seen a tremendous increase in popularity, and it's received some bad reviews, especially for women. This is largely because many women haven't been taught how to cycle their low carbohydrate diets with their hormones. In my book Fast Like a Girl, I extensively map out how women of all ages do exactly that. I strongly feel menopausal women need to do the ketogenic diet differently. What I have mapped out for you in this chapter is a beautiful way to get the amazing benefits of going keto while still preserving your gut microbiome and balancing your hormones. The best of both worlds.

THE 28-DAY HORMONE RESET

Day 1 to 11: Ketobiotic diet with your choice of fast.

Day 12 to 14: Estrogen-building foods with intermittent fasting.

Day 15 to 21: Ketobiotic diet with your choice of fast.

Day 21 to 28: Progesterone-building foods with intermittent fasting.

CHAPTER 8

●●●●●●●●●●●●●●●●●●●

Meet Your Estrobolome

I've got good news and bad news. The good news? Everything I have just taught you about eating, fasting, and your hormones is applicable to your human cells. The bad news? By current estimates human cells make up only around 50 percent of who you are. The rest of you is bacteria, fungi, parasites, and viruses. Sound disgusting? Well, it's not. These microbes can work miracles. The fabulous thing about these microbes is you can feed them healthy food, and they will get stronger and more powerful. In this chapter, I want to show you exactly how to power up these miraculous microbes.

First, let me introduce you to your microbiome. *Microbiome* is the term used to explain all the amazing microbes you have living in and on you. You have trillions of different microbes that are on your skin, in your gut, surrounding every organ, and living in your vaginal and nasal mucous membranes. You even have a whole world of good microbes in your mouth. If you are like most, you have been taught to fear microbes.

We live in a world that is obsessed with killing bacteria. We have an antibacterial solution for just about everything. But what we have forgotten to keep in mind is that we have bad bacteria and good bacteria. The good bacteria make some incredible chemicals for us, like serotonin, which keeps us happy, or GABA, which calms our brain. We have bacteria that control our immune system and regulate our blood sugar and speed up our metabolism. We even have a whole set of bacteria that helps us remove harmful estrogens from our bodies. Bacteria are our friends, yet we've only been taught how to kill them. It's time to change that. I want to teach you how to nurture and grow these amazing bacteria so that you get all the health benefits they can offer.

There are two ways to nurture good bacteria. First, you need to stop destroying them. I will walk you through some of the most damaging habits that are killing these good little guys. Second, you must feed them. Don't kill them and keep them fed: it's that simple. Think of these good bacteria as a pet that lives inside of you. You want to create an environment where they can thrive and grow.

What Destroys Good Bacteria?

This antibiotic-rich world is not only killing off the bad guys; it's destroying the good ones, too. If you want to nurture these good bacteria, you will need to stop the influx of bug killers. We call these antibacterials. Look at your personal world right now. Where might you be getting a daily dose of antibacterials?

Start by asking yourself:

- Am I using antibacterial soaps?
- Do I brush or rinse my mouth with antibacterial toothpaste or mouthwash?

- Am I eating meats with antibiotics in them?
- How many rounds of antibiotics have I been on in my life?

The greater your antibiotic exposure, the fewer good bacteria you will likely have. One round of prescribed oral antibiotics can kill up to 90 percent of your good bacteria, massively restructuring the diversity of your gut. This is a huge problem in our world today. We have little respect for these good microbes. I have consulted with thousands of women who have been on more antibiotics than they can count. These same women suffer from depression, anxiety, and insomnia or have been diagnosed with multiple auto-immune conditions. Missing these good bacteria means missing the chemicals that keep you healthy and happy. This is such an important concept to grasp that I want to make sure it is the first task you take on in resetting your microbiome. Stop the influx of antibiotics.

Once you have accomplished this, the next step I want you to take is to minimize the toxins coming into your body. This applies both to toxins that go in your mouth and those you put on your skin. I dive into toxins in more detail in the next chapter, but for now, I want you to understand that the higher your toxic load, the fewer good bacteria you will have.

The easiest way to stop toxifying your gut is to stop eating fake foods. Not all food is created equal. There are real foods that nature made and fake foods that man made. Real foods like fruits and vegetables don't typically destroy your gut microbiome. They feed it. Man-made foods like preservatives, artificial sweeteners, food colorings, food additives, or hydrogenated oils will make it difficult for your good bacteria to thrive. Here is a list of foods I highly recommend you stay away from on a regular basis, as they destroy your happy bugs:

- Monosodium glutamate (MSG)
- Artificial food coloring
- Sodium nitrite
- Guar gum
- High-fructose corn syrup
- Artificial sweeteners
- Trans fats (like partially hydrogenated oils, canola oil, or vegetable oil)

You'll find most fake foods in the center aisles of your grocery store. They usually have a long shelf life and little nutritional value. I recommend you shop the perimeter of the market as much as possible. This is where you will find the more perishable foods that may not last as long in your refrigerator but will do wonders for your good bacteria.

One final thought on the killing of your good bacteria: your microbial world is incredibly intelligent, and bacteria communicate with each other often. This is especially true with your gut microbiome and your skin microbiome. Whatever you put in your gut will come out of your skin. We see this with acne. The gut bacteria have trouble breaking down dairy, so it gets pushed out through the skin. We also see this the other way around. What you put on your skin can affect your gut. If you are consistently putting toxic chemicals or antibacterial soaps on your skin, it will have an adverse effect on the microbes in your gut. This is such an important concept that in my Microbiome Reset protocol I recommend you use probiotic-rich lotions like Derma Colonizer by Systemic Formulas to keep your skin microbiome happy—thus supporting a healthy gut microbiome.

What to Feed Your Good Bacteria

Now that you have an idea of how to stop the destruction of your good bacteria, let's talk about how you can feed these happy critters. There are three categories of food that your good microbes like to eat: polyphenol, probiotic, and prebiotic. In Michael Pollan's book *In Defense of Food*, he states, "Eat food, not too much, mostly plants." He is spot on. I couldn't agree with him more. Plants are fuel for your good microbiome. The more you eat them, the happier your good bacteria will be. Polyphenol and prebiotic foods will help you grow the good bacteria you already have, while probiotic-rich foods will add good bacteria to your gut. You need a balance of these three food categories on a daily basis.

My favorite polyphenol foods are:

- Cloves
- Olives
- Dark chocolate
- Berries
- Raw nuts
- Red wine

My favorite prebiotic foods are:

- Chia seeds
- Hemp seeds
- Flax seeds

My favorite probiotic-rich foods are:

- Sauerkraut
- Kimchi

- Probiotic-rich yogurts
- Probiotic-rich drinks (kombucha, kefir water)
- Raw dairy kefir

Unfortunately, we don't have specific research on how much of these foods you should be eating every day. But keep in mind that diversity of these foods is key. In a recent interview I did with Dr. Terry Wahls, author of *The Wahls Protocol*, she talked about how important the diversity of your plant intake can be. Dr. Wahls has an incredible story. She alleviated her symptoms of multiple sclerosis through diet. I highly recommend you check out her TED Talk called "Minding Your Mitochondria." What struck me the most about our conversation is her commitment to getting over 200 different plants into her diet over a one-year period. Try it; it's a fun challenge. I loved this idea so much, I dedicate a whole day of my Forever Young Reset program to plant diversity. On this day, I have people fast for 24 hours to start intestinal stem cell production and follow that up with 15 different plants to feed their good gut microbiome.

Meet Your Estrobolome

All of your good bacteria serve different purposes. Some make neurotransmitters, others protect you against high cholesterol, and yet others help you breakdown B vitamins in your food so they are more readily absorbed. These bacteria are busy. There is a group of bacteria that will be especially helpful to you on your menopause journey. They're called your estrobolome. This group of helpful bacteria does two things for you: break down toxic estrogens and activate helpful estrogen. These are the bacteria you want to grow.

Your estrobolome is made up of a group of over 60 bacteria. When these bacteria are thriving, your hormones will thrive. Microbes in the estrobolome also produce beta-glucuronidase. This is a key enzyme you need to ensure that the little bit of healthy estrogen you produce in your menopause years gets activated into your cells. The more beta-glucuronidase you have, the less good estrogen is excreted out of the body.

Remember, you have good estrogen and bad estrogen. If you want to thrive in your menopause years, you will want to be sure to have plenty of the good and are capable of breaking down the bad. When your gut microbes are out of balance, beta-glucuronidase activity may be altered. This dysbiosis can lead to an imbalance in estrogen. Excess estrogen is the source of many pathologies and chronic diseases.

Common signs that your estrobolome is out of balance:

- Bloating and digestive upset
- Acne
- Low libido
- Heavy, light, or irregular periods
- Tender, swollen, and/or fibrocystic breasts
- Headaches
- Weight gain
- Hot flashes
- Mood swings
- Polycystic ovarian syndrome (PCOS)
- Cancers of the breast or ovaries

The simplest way to understand your estrobolome is with an at-home stool test. The test I recommend is called

Gut Zoomer by Vibrant Wellness. Not only will this stool test tell you which pathogens you need to kill, but it will tell you if you have the right balance of good bacteria. This is incredibly helpful if you are trying to balance hormones, lose weight, stop chronic pain, or bring happiness back to your brain.

Two of my favorite bacteria in the estrobolome are *Lactobacillus reuteri* and *Lactobacillus rhamnosus*. Keep an eye out for these bacteria when you are buying probiotics. These are the estrogen-balancing bacteria. They are both present in my favorite supplement for menopausal women: Femicrine by Systemic Formulas.

One of the ways you can nurture these two bacteria is by adding more phytoestrogens into your diet. Some of the most helpful phytoestrogens that support your estrobolome are:

- Black cohosh
- Broccoli
- Carrots
- Chaste tree berry
- Organic coffee
- Dong quai
- Evening primrose
- Legumes (beans, peas, peanuts)
- Licorice root
- Oranges
- Red clover
- Organic soy (tofu, tempeh, miso, soy milk)

Keep Your Liver Happy

Your liver is another organ that breaks down estrogen. Your liver, gallbladder, and small intestine work closely together. If you take amazing care of your gut microbiome but put extra stress on your liver, you still end up with hormones out of balance.

Some of the best practices for optimal liver function are:

- Minimize liver stressors like alcohol, medications, fried foods, and sugary desserts.
- Increase cruciferous vegetables like brussels sprouts, broccoli, and cauliflower.
- Use castor oil packs (3x per week).
- Try a coffee enema (1x per week).
- Take supplements to get key nutrients to a liver that may be struggling.

Purge Your Pathogens

One final note about your gut microbe that needs to be addressed: in addition to being deficient in good bacteria, you may also need to kill off pathogens. Pathogens are the bullies of your gut microbiome. They hijack the terrain inside the gut and make it difficult for the good guys to grow. They can also control your cravings and give you unpleasant symptoms.

Pathogens come in all different forms: parasites, viruses, bacteria, and fungi. The pathogen that I see harm hormonal balance the most is *Candida albicans*. This is a fungus that makes you crave sugar, refined carbohydrates, and alcohol. It can give you brain fog, make you hold on to weight, and contributes to vaginal yeast infections.

There are several ways to understand if you have this pathogen hanging out in your gut. Cravings are a good start. My patients who have uncontrollable sugar cravings usually have *Candida*. Its preferred fuel source is sugar, so in order to keep itself alive, it makes you crave it. Head symptoms like brain fog or ringing in the ears are other telltale signs, as are any of the classic yeast symptoms, such as rashes, itchy skin, or recurring vaginal infections.

Look at your tongue first thing in the morning. If there is a white or yellow coat on your tongue, that too can be a sign of *Candida*. This coat especially shows up while you are fasting. A stool test like Gut Zoomer will also confirm if *Candida* or any other pathogen is present in your gut.

Reset Your Microbiome

As you can see, there is a lot to your gut microbiome. It's a fragile and complicated system, but if you take amazing care of it, then it will serve you well. Because of the importance of your microbiome to your overall health, I wanted to leave you with the Microbiome Reset protocol that I put all my patients on. Along with the other recommendations I have talked about in this chapter, here are three major additions I would make to your daily routine.

Change your toothpaste.

I highly recommend a prebiotic toothpaste that will feed the good bacteria in your mouth. These good bacteria will help you break down your food so that you don't send undigested food into your stomach. If you are missing this good mouth bacteria, you will send food on to the stomach that is not predigested. This can often allow undigested food to ferment in your stomach, causing *Candida* to grow even stronger. The brand I recommend to my patients is Revitin.

Use a probiotic lotion.

Remember the skin-gut connection? When you get out of the shower, I want you to put a probiotic lotion on your abdomen. This starts to get helpful bacteria moving from your skin to your gut. Be sure to get some of this lotion in your belly button as there is a placental connection from your belly button to your liver. There are a lot of good probiotic lotions on the market. The one I like best is Skin Colonizer by Systemic Formulas.

Replace missing microbes.

Getting key protective bacteria into your gut on a daily basis is important. But the soil most of our food is grown in is depleted of minerals and helpful bacteria. Because of that, I recommend a supplement called Ion Gut Support by Intelligence of Nature, which helps replenish key missing bacteria that used to be in our soils years ago. Ion Biome was created by Dr. Zach Bush, an endocrinologist who realized that many of his patients were ill because of missing microbes. He discovered that the soils our food grows in are missing key protective good bacteria that used to be in our soils decades ago. When he reintroduced these bacteria back into his patients' guts, they started to heal. Under the microscope, Dr. Bush and his team noticed that these missing bacteria sealed up a leaky gut within 20 minutes of ingesting them. Once a leaky gut is sealed up, toxins no longer get into the bloodstream. Because of the healing power of these missing microbes, this is the one supplement that I recommend all my patients stay on. They even have a nasal spray that will help provide the protective bacteria for your nasal mucous membranes.

Hopefully, you feel like there is a lot you can do to support your microbiome. The microbiome is a new frontier. Every day, researchers are discovering more about just how helpful bacteria can be to our bodies. You got this. Resetting your microbiome can be fun.

MARY'S STORY

When Mary hit her late 40s, she experienced excruciating migraines, insomnia, and excessive hair loss, which dramatically impacted her work and personal life. She was right in the center of her menopause journey with no understanding of how to get well. Life was crashing down on her. She became incredibly stressed out, tired, and unhappy, and was desperately searching for answers.

She had had chronic fatigue in her early 30s due to adrenal, thyroid, and digestive imbalances. She had spent a large part of her 30s healing those conditions. Then she hit her mid-40s and all those symptoms reappeared. She was already eating a healthy Paleo anti-inflammatory diet, had made significant lifestyle changes, and had a dedicated yoga and meditation practice.

One of the superpowers that Mary has is that she is incredibly tenacious and willing to be proactive, especially when it comes to her health. She had been to numerous holistic doctors and was willing to do anything that would get her well. The discouraging part for her was despite all her efforts, she still wasn't getting well. Her sleepless nights and excessive hair loss were causing her so much anxiety and stress she was desperate for a new solution.

She read my first book, *The Reset Factor*, and resonated with my customized multi-therapeutic approach to healing the body. She then reached out to me for a health consultation. When I sat down with her for the first time, I had one mission: finally help Mary get to the root cause of her symptoms.

The first thing I did with Mary was get her a series of functional medicine tests so I could see why she wasn't healing. The tests revealed that she had a leaky gut, adrenal fatigue, and low progesterone and estrogen levels. With these results, I created a game plan for her, combining several of my favorite healing tools. Quickly, Mary regained her health—no more migraines, sleepless nights, anxiety, exhaustion, or hair loss. A large part of Mary's healing needed to happen in her gut. Once I found the right path for her gut, her hormones improved as well.

It's been two years since I first tested Mary. She now has amazing energy and has been able to fulfill a dream of hers this past year: traveling to Bali and Italy with no health complications. She now knows that all healing roads for her lead to her gut. If she wants to stay her best, she just needs to use the tools I taught her to keep her gut in good shape. Not only does she feel better than she has in decades, but she is also back in control of health. That's an awesome place to be.

Next Steps to Resetting Your Microbiome

- Minimize the amount of antibacterials that you touch or ingest.
- Avoid toxic fake foods packed with synthetic chemicals and harmful oils.
- Add in polyphenol, prebiotic, and probiotic-rich foods.
- Support your liver.
- Nurture your estrobolome.
- Test and purge any pathogens.
- Follow the daily microbiome reset.

It's been so inspiring to serve health from a functional medicine perspective for the past 23 years. So much has changed in how we view our health. We used to think our health was determined only by our genes. Then we learned about the science of epigenetics and how our lifestyle can turn genes on and off. Then in 2007, the Human Microbiome Project was launched and how we look at genes changed one more time. This six-year project discovered that bacteria on us and in us have a massive effect on our gene expression. The Human Microbiome Project also gave us a deep respect for the helpful bacteria that can have a powerful effect on metabolism, lower cholesterol, produce neurotransmitters, and regulate our immune systems. Bottom line: we need to take better care of these bacteria. Since the birth of the Human Microbiome Project, more and more research keeps surfacing on just how miraculous bacteria can be for our health. It's an exciting time. Once you get the hang of feeding these helpful microbes, you will see just how great they can make you feel.

CHAPTER 9

•••••••••••••••••••

Is Detox More Important Than Lifestyle?

We live in the most toxic time in human history. In the past 60 years, over 87,000 new chemicals have entered into our environment. These toxins have entered into our food, water, and soils. They are on our furniture, in our beauty products, and woven into the fabric of our clothes. We are even exposed to toxins in the dental chair, with our yearly flu shot, and in medications. Many of these toxins, called carcinogens, are known to cause cancer, and others, called neurotoxins, damage nervous tissue. These toxins get stored in the tissues of your body, damaging healthy tissue. These toxins are bioaccumulating at a faster rate than ever before, and the human body struggles because of it.

No one struggles more from this increased toxin load than the menopausal woman. Let me tell you why. Dramatic shifts in your hormones during the menopausal years stimulate the tissues in your body to release toxins. For example, lead lives in your bones and often will get released during your menopausal years. This adds to a menopausal women's hormonal nightmare because as lead is released it will mobilize to another part of the body. Toxins love to accumulate in nervous tissue and fat. Your brain is made up of both of these. This makes the brain extremely vulnerable to the bioaccumulation of toxins. But remember, you are miraculously designed. You came with a protective barrier surrounding your brain to protect it from harmful chemicals. It's called your blood-brain barrier. It protects your brain with the exception of three areas: the hypothalamus, the pituitary, and pineal gland. These are the areas that control all hormonal production. Once toxins settle here, your whole hormonal system will be thrown off.

It doesn't matter how clean your lifestyle is, detoxing your brain is key. It's a path back to restoring balance to your already declining hormones. This is exactly what happened to me. When menopause hit me hard, I lived as close to a clean and healthy lifestyle as one could live. But I still had massive hot flashes, trouble sleeping, mood swings, trouble with mental clarity, and low energy. The piece that I didn't address was my toxic load. It wasn't until I learned how to detox these environmental toxins that I got my life back. In this chapter, I will teach you which toxins you need to look for and what you can do to properly detox them out of your body.

When it comes to detoxing, the first questions to ask yourself are "Which toxins are affecting me the most?" and "How the heck am I going to get rid of them?" The hard part of managing your toxic load is understanding the vast amount of toxins you are exposed to on a daily basis. I've tried to understand the more than 87,000 chemicals that have been introduced into our environment in the past 60 years. It has led me down rabbit holes of research trying to get to the bottom of which toxins are the most harmful. But instead of boring you with long lists of chemicals, I have broken them down into three major categories: forever chemicals, endocrine disruptors, and heavy metals.

Forever Chemicals

PFAs, which are per- and polyfluoroalkyl substances, comprise a classification of over 5,000 chemicals that are incredibly persistent in our environment and can accumulate quickly in our bodies. PFAs have been linked to lowered immune function, thyroid conditions, kidney disease, elevated cholesterol, and reproductive problems. What is perhaps the scariest thing about these chemicals is they are designated as possible carcinogens and won't leave your body easily. Studies show that PFAs have a half-life of 92 years in our environment and 8 years in the human body. Can you see why they are being called forever chemicals? These nasty toxins plan on hanging around for a long time.

PFAs don't just affect one part of your body; they can have a systemic effect as well. According to the Environmental Working Group, the immune system is particularly vulnerable to forever chemicals and new studies suggest there is a strong connection between PFA exposure and suppressed immune function, lower vaccine effectiveness, and greater risk of autoimmune diseases.[7]

Think about this for a moment. Have you ever been at work where there is a virulent cold going around? Some people catch the cold while others don't. Why is that? What if your toxic load plays a part in how strong your immune reaction will be?

What about the rise in autoimmune conditions? Studies are now proving that genetics contribute to only 30 percent of all autoimmune conditions. Seventy percent of autoimmune conditions are due to environmental toxins.[8] Women have a higher incidence and prevalence of autoimmune diseases than men, and 85 percent or more patients with multiple autoimmune diseases are female. These autoimmune conditions often show up at times of sweeping hormonal changes such as menopause.[9]

How do you go about avoiding these chemicals? Well, unfortunately, it's nearly impossible to avoid them completely. They are in your drinking water, food packaging, upholstery, mattresses, carpet treatments, Teflon pans, and even your clothing.

There are a few smart steps you can take to reduce your exposure:

- Remove your Teflon pans and replace them with cast iron.
- Avoid prepacked foods that come in Styrofoam, plastics, or cardboard to-go containers.
- When purchasing furniture, seek out organic materials.
- Invest in a reverse-osmosis water filter.

Endocrine Disruptors

Endocrine disrupting chemicals (EDCs) are ubiquitous in our environment as well. You may have heard of endocrine disruptors in association with hormonal cancers like breast or ovarian. But these chemicals don't have to give you a cancer diagnosis to cause you problems. They can throw your estrogen and progesterone balance off, leaving you with hair loss, hot flashes, anxiety, insomnia, and weight gain for no reason.

The most common endocrine disruptors are:

- Bisphenol A (BPA) plastics
- Polychlorinated biphenyls (PCBs)
- Dichlorodiphenyltrichloroethane (DDT)
- Dioxins
- Pesticides
- Parabens
- Phthalates
- Heavy metals

Endocrine-disrupting chemicals are known to block the receptor sites for hormones. Receptor sites are the openings into a cell that allow hormones into the cell to activate a specific action in your body. For example, your T3 hormone goes into cells and activates metabolism. If a toxin is blocking a receptor site, that hormone can't get in and you will be left with a slow metabolism.

Remember how the brain sends a signal to certain endocrine glands to secrete hormones? If your brain is healthy and the endocrine gland is functioning well, you still can be exhibiting signs of hormonal imbalance due to blocked receptor sites. This is a common scenario with thyroid symptoms.

Many women experience symptoms of a thyroid problem, yet their doctors will look at their blood work and say they are fine. Why don't they feel fine, then? Or worse yet, many women are put on thyroid medication but still feel horrible. If this is you, there is a good chance your thyroid problems are a not a gland issue but rather one of blocked receptor sites.

Minimizing your exposure to endocrine disruptors will make a huge difference in your hormonal health. The biggest strides you can make in lowering your EDCs are the following.

Scan your beauty products.

Think Dirty is an app developed by the Breast Cancer Prevention Partners that will let you scan your beauty products to see if they contain carcinogens, hormone disruptors, or allergens. I recommend that my patients scan everything that goes on their skin or hair. You want those products to score a three or less on the Think Dirty scale.

Eat organic.

Eating organic is not just for hippies anymore. It's for anyone who wants to stay healthy and prevent disease. Not only are pesticides known carcinogens, but they block receptor sites for hormones as well.

An endocrine gland that is especially vulnerable to pesticides is your thyroid. Pesticides can block receptor sites for thyroid hormones and destroy healthy thyroid tissue. The thyroid is often called the canary in the coal mine. When you see your thyroid gland malfunction, it's a sign your toxic load is high.

Organic foods are everywhere now. If costs are of concern, the first place you want to start is with your meat. There are more pesticides in the animals we eat than what is sprayed on our fruits and vegetables. The next step is to follow the guidelines of the Environmental Working Group's Dirty Dozen and Clean Fifteen. This is a powerful list that notes which fruits and vegetables should be organic and which ones are not as heavily sprayed (i.e., it's okay to buy conventional). In my house, we eat a lot of avocados, which are on the Clean Fifteen list. Since organic avocados are twice the cost of conventional ones, we often buy the conventional ones.

Toss the plastic.

BPA plastics are also destroying your hormones. Not only are they damaging to all your endocrine glands, but they also block receptor sites and settle into your brain. If you are still using plastic bags or plastic containers for your food, now is the time to stop. The chemicals in plastics leach out into your food and contribute to your menopause symptoms.

In my household, we use glass containers, both for storing leftovers and for all our water bottles. This was an easy switch, and it took me just one day of going into the kitchen and tossing out anything that seemed to contain plastics. It's a worthy endeavor that will save you many sleepless nights and a few hot flashes.

Train your toxic lens.

I want you to start looking at everything you eat, drink, breathe, or touch through a toxic lens. Ask yourself, "Are there chemicals in here? Can I find a natural version of this?" I call these lateral changes. You are just swapping out a toxic version for a natural one. A great example of something you can easily swap out is air fresheners. Commercial fresheners for your car and home are known endocrine disruptors.[10] Can you replace them with essential oils and diffusers?

What about prepacked food? What can you make yourself? For example, microwave popcorn is massively toxic. I buy organic popcorn kernels to make at home. Not only do I get skip the EDCs and forever chemicals, I get to drizzle some grass-fed butter onto my popcorn.

Once you start looking at everything through a toxic lens, it will become second nature to choose the healthier, nontoxic items. Awareness is the first step. It is like shopping for a car. Once you know the car you want, you spot it everywhere on the road. The same will happen with toxins. You will start not only identifying toxic items, but you will also develop taste buds that tell you if a food is fresh or toxic. I promise you, it's a muscle you can train. Once you train it, your long-term health will greatly improve.

This is what happened to Terri, a 54-year-old postmenopausal patient of mine who struggled with her hormones. Even though she hadn't had a period in over three years, she still experienced hot flashes, had trouble sleeping, and no matter how hard she tried, couldn't lose weight.

I ran a DUTCH test on her and discovered that her harmful estrogen metabolites were extremely high. She was new to understanding her toxic environment. I asked her to look at the toxins she might be continually exposed to every day. At that time, Terri was not eating organic, many of her household cleaners and beauty products were highly toxic, and she was on the go a lot, often eating out of plastic-packaged foods. Yet she was committed to her health and knew she needed to change.

She spent several months undoing her toxic habits. With each major change to her toxic environment her symptoms improved. Within a year's time, her hot flashes were gone, she started to finally lose weight, and she was sleeping again. She was doing so well we decided to run another DUTCH test. Her harmful estrogen metabolites had lowered. Removing toxins from her world was lifesaving. I'm so proud of her.

Heavy Metals

Heavy metals are a menopausal woman's nightmare. Many metals like lead and mercury live in your tissues and are released into your bloodstream at times of hormonal swings: puberty, pregnancy, and menopause. Once in the bloodstream, they will often go to the brain and wreak havoc on the parts of your brain that regulate your hormones.

Heavy metals are the most harmful of all the toxins. They can be the major reason you are losing your memory, feeling depressed and irritable, and not sleeping. Many of these metals you unknowingly accumulated years ago. In some cases, your heavy metal load was passed down to you by your mother when you were in the womb. For some of you, your metal load is high because of generational exposure from your mother or grandmother. I know this was the case in my menopausal journey.

Because heavy metals are released from stored tissues, they can sneak up on you. I know a menopausal woman is dealing with heavy metal toxicity when she says to me, "Out of nowhere, I started having trouble sleeping," or "All my old tricks for losing weight are not working anymore," or "I feel sorry for my poor husband because I am just so irritable and easily agitated." Those are classic signs heavy metals are being released.

Two of the most common metals contributing to your menopausal roller coaster are lead and mercury.

Lead

I have tested thousands of patients for heavy metals and not one has come back free of lead. Lead lives in your bones. During menopause, it will be released into your bloodstream, irritating nerves, weakening bones, and slowing down your memory. I can't tell you the number of cases I have seen of menopausal women with high lead that are osteoporotic, experiencing chronic pain, depressed, and starting to struggle to retrieve their words. These are classic signs of lead toxicity. I think of lead as a suppressant. It slows down thoughts, robs you of joy, weakens your bones, and leaves you with dull chronic pain.

Mercury

Mercury, on the other hand, is excitatory. It is the metal that makes you feel agitated, irritable, and restless, and will keep you up at night. It's more of a stimulant. Anxiety is already high in menopausal women due to declining levels of progesterone, but if you add a high mercury load to that, you've got yourself one irritable menopausal woman.

There are ways to minimize your exposure to toxic heavy metals. Some of the more common places you are currently exposed to heavy metals are:

- Dentist (amalgam fillings and crowns)
- Flu shots
- Fish
- Remodeling an old home that used lead paint
- Beauty products, especially lipstick
- Ceramic dishware
- Drinking water

• Vegetables and fruit grown in soils with heavy metals

You *can* get these toxins out. But fasting, stimulating autophagy, juice cleansing, or colon cleanses will not do the trick. There are four specific steps I recommend you take when you detox heavy metals and environmental toxins.

1. **Know your toxic load.**

    Since toxins live in stored tissues, it's hard to know exactly how high your toxic load may be. Blood and hair tests will only tell us what is currently circulating in your system. They won't tell you what is stored in bone, fat, or nervous tissue. This is why we recommend to our patients a provoked heavy metal test. This is a urine test where you take a provoking agent like DMSA to pull metals out of the stored tissues and move them to your urine for measurement.

    Testing your toxic load can help you create a plan of action. Without this plan, you may never know how much you need to detox and for how long.

2. **Open up your detox pathways.**

    Remember that you are dealing with synthetic, man-made chemicals. Before you launch into any type of deep detox, you want to make sure the organs of detoxification are healthy and ready for the job. The major detoxification organs are your liver, gut, kidneys, skin, and lymph system.

Some strategies that open up detox pathways and support these organs are:

Dry Brushing: Dry brushing is a technique using a natural organic brush on your skin. It helps detoxify by increasing blood circulation and promoting lymph flow/ drainage. Dry brushing can unclog pores in the exfoliation process. It also stimulates your nervous system, which can make you feel invigorated afterward. I love dry brushing.

Infrared Saunas: Infrared saunas are different from your regular gym sauna. Infrared light heats your cells up from the inside out, much like a fever does. When the cells heat up from the inside out, they can burn out infections, release toxins, and restore the cell's ability to breathe.

Coffee Enemas: As daunting as a coffee enema may sound, it's a life-changing experience for so many of my patients. Coffee enemas are exactly as they sound. Instead of water used as an enema, you use coffee. When coffee is administered to your body in this fashion, it will dilate the common bile duct, which is the pathway for the liver to push out toxins.

Red Light Therapy: Red light is healing. We use red light all the time in my clinic to stimulate cellular healing. When you put red light into a cell, it heals the outer cell membrane and activates your mitochondria. The mitochondria are the part of the cell that initiates detox within the cell.

PEMF: Think of your mitochondria as the battery of your cells. If your battery is low, your cells will stay inflamed and toxins will not be able to get out. Pulsed electromagnetic field therapy, or PEMF, sends healthy electromagnetic frequencies into cells that power up the mitochondria so that they can detox again.

Hyperbaric Oxygen Chambers: Oxygen is also helpful to your cells as you detox. As we age, our cells' ability to pull in oxygen becomes compromised. Hyperbaric oxygen is compressed oxygen that allows oxygen to easily enter the cell. Once your cells have more oxygen, the mitochondria will heal, allowing them to push toxins out of the cells effortlessly.

Supplementation: Remember methylation? Well, many nutrients are necessary for methylation to occur within the cells. Nutrients like B vitamins and CoQ10. When we are working with a patient to open up their detox pathways, we use a supplement called MORS by Systemic Formulas. This supplement supports a proper methylation process and helps your cells detox.

These are pivotal tools I use in our clinic to help our patients have an easy time detoxing. The science behind many of the techniques described here is in Chapter 11.

3. **Remove toxins from your body first.**

    Once you grasp how toxins contribute to your menopause symptoms, I promise you will feel compelled to jump into a brain detox right away. Everyone wants the toxins out of their brain immediately. I get it. When your brain is free of toxins, your menopause symptoms will dramatically change.

    Remember: when toxins are removed from your brain, they will filter through your liver, gut, kidneys, and lymph system. I highly recommend you detox those organs first. Otherwise, it's like trying to empty your full kitchen trash can into your overly full curbside trash can. The toxins will just spill over into other tissues.

Some of the best ways to detox the body are:

- Increase your glutathione levels either through supplementation or cruciferous vegetables.
- Improve cellular membrane function by increasing good fats.
- Use binders like activated charcoal, zeolites, or DMSA.
- Improve methylation through supplementation or increasing sulfur-rich foods.

4. Remove toxins from the brain.

This is where you get your life back. This is where you start to feel normal again. Detoxing feels like someone took a magic wand to my brain. I've done so many brain detoxes now that the minute I hop on one, my brain instantly feels joyful, clear, and focused again. There are several strategies I find helpful for brain detoxing:

Increase ketone production: Remember, ketones are what you naturally produce when you fast. If you are brain detoxing, fasting for longer periods to increase ketone production can be helpful.

Mega-dose on minerals: Your brain needs minerals to function normally. A simple depletion of zinc can cause massive depression for a person. Toxins often sit in the receptor sites for minerals, so as you remove those toxins your brain will need more minerals to function normally. I highly recommend that you increase your mineral consumption when you are on a brain detox. The mineral supplement we recommend is called MIN by Systemic Formulas.

Supplement with alpha-lipoic acid like that used in Brain DTX: One of the challenges we have with detoxing the brain is getting past the blood-brain barrier. Few nutrients can cross this powerful barrier. The supplement we recommend for brain detoxing is called Brain DTX. It is made up of a nutrient called alpha-lipoic acid that can go deep into parts of your brain and shake toxins loose.

Supplement with binders DMSA and Zeolites like those used in Cytodetox®: The key to all detoxing is using binders. Binders will hold on to toxins as they exit the cells. This is incredibly important so that toxins don't get reabsorbed. When detoxing the brain, our favorite binder is Cytodetox because it has the strongest ability to magnetize metals.

Schedule weekly hyperbaric oxygen chamber sessions: As toxins exit your brain cells, driving oxygen into the cells can be healing. In our clinic, we recommend hyperbaric oxygen chambers for patients as they move through the brain detox process. More information on hyperbaric oxygen can be found in Chapter 11.

Schedule weekly chiropractic adjustments: You might know chiropractic as a cure for back and neck pain, but current research shows that it does a lot more than that. We now know that chiropractic adjustment improves the flow of cerebral spinal fluid in and out of the brain. Cerebral spinal fluid is responsible for detoxing. A chiropractic adjustment also prompts the brain to move from a place of fight-or-flight into a place of hope and possibility. Our patients who incorporate weekly chiropractic adjustments into their brain detoxes heal quicker with fewer detox symptoms.

I always feel like a downer when I talk toxins. I know that it is a huge task to understand and detox these chemicals. I tried solving my menopausal roller coaster with lifestyle changes alone. It didn't work. Once I understood toxins and committed to regular detoxes, I felt like myself again. I see this scenario is also true for countless other women. Relief from turbulent menopause symptoms is in the detox.

RACHEL'S STORY

For 18 years, Rachel's identity was wrapped up in the label of hypothyroid disease, which she'd been diagnosed with after having some pretty nasty symptoms that made it hard for her to function normally. Her days were filled with unrelenting fatigue, depression, terrible acne, brittle hair and skin, and weight gain that would not cease despite clean foods and exercise. The hardest part for Rachel was that she was out of answers and couldn't find a doctor who believed there was a way out of this nightmare.

Rachel decided to take her health into her own hands. She started to learn all that she could about the causes of hypothyroidism. One day, while she was down a rabbit hole of thyroid information, she came across a podcast where I was interviewed by Katie Wells, The Wellness Mama, on generational toxicity. A light bulb went off for her. No one had connected toxins to her sluggish thyroid. Maybe this was the missing piece to her health puzzle. She reached out to me for a health consultation. I dove into her health history and found out that Rachel's toxic load was extremely high. Detoxing heavy metals was the missing piece.

One thing that is incredibly important to me is that my patients understand how to detox properly. I get so many patients who have been ill advised on how to remove toxins the right way, slowly and efficiently. Rachel's toxic load was so high that I wanted to make sure she knew how to pull toxins out so she could keep detoxing for years to come.

We have been working together now for over a year. She has lost 55 pounds, her hair has stopped falling out, she feels vibrant and energetic, her dark moods have lifted, and her skin is glowing. She has become so empowered by what she has learned about detoxing that she's gone on to test her three daughters' heavy metal loads as well. I have been working with her to create a detox plan for them that will ensure they stay healthy before a diagnosis of hypothyroidism appears.

Rachel's story is such a powerful reminder that knowledge is power. When you know why your body isn't functioning well, you can create a plan to heal it. For Rachel, the root cause of her thyroid breaking down was heavy metal toxicity, specifically lead. The detox journey has given Rachel her life back. More importantly, she now has the knowledge and tools to keep her thyroid healthy for life.

There are so many reasons I love Rachel's healing story. But perhaps what I love the most is how Rachel listened to that inner voice that said, "You can heal. You don't have to accept this diagnosis." Because she listened to that voice and took healing into her hands, she now has the energy to be present for her family, a reignited passion to give to others, and a brain that no longer fails her. Hope has been restored. As Rachel so often beautifully states, "When you have hope, you can conquer the world."

Next Steps to Detoxing Your Life

- Scan your beauty products.
- Commit to eating organic whenever possible.
- Toss the plastic.
- Train your toxic lens.
- Know your toxic load.
- Open up your detox pathways.
- Pull toxins from your body.
- Pull toxins from your brain.

I have spent countless hours studying and applying different natural healing techniques. Few things have been as miraculous to a person's life as detoxing. We are living in such a toxic time, and our toxin buckets are filling up fast. Knowing how to detox properly is lifesaving.

Your cells cannot heal when they are packed with toxins. If you have tried everything to heal yourself and feel like nothing is working, it's time to detox. I promise you that miracles happen when you remove these chemicals from your body. You will heal better, feel better, and function at a higher level of health than you know to be possible.

CHAPTER 10

Stop the Rushing Woman's Syndrome

A few years back, one of my colleagues and friends recommended a book to me called *Rushing Woman's Syndrome* by Dr. Libby Weaver. When I first heard the name of the book, I thought, "Wow, do I ever need to read that!" Since I was truly a rushing woman, I never made time to read it. Pretty ironic, right?

But my friend kept reminding me. Finally, I bought the book and took it on vacation with me. Was she right! It was life-changing. Within reading the first couple of pages, I could see my overscheduled life was exacerbating my already-declining sex hormones.

As I dove deeper into understanding stress and its effects on sex hormones, I realized that my busy, overscheduled life was keeping my brain in a state of fight-or-flight. Once my brain perceived it was in a crisis, it shut down sex hormone production. This is a recipe for disaster for a woman going through menopause. I realized that just because I am a skilled rushing woman doesn't mean it's in my hormonal best interest to keep rushing.

For weeks, I contemplated that thought. At this point, I had already implemented a lot of the changes I've discussed in this book. I had built a fasting lifestyle. I ate for my cycle (when it showed up). I had already done several deep detoxes. And I was diligent about feeding my microbiome. I was doing everything possible to minimize the menopausal roller coaster that had begun in my early 40s. It was working for me. Yet I still felt like there was a piece missing to my hormone puzzle. I still had a few surges of symptoms like insomnia, irritability, and an occasional hot flash.

Could it be that the last piece to my hormonal puzzle was to stop rushing? The only way I was going to know for sure how my overscheduled life was affecting me was with a DUTCH hormone test. I ran one on myself. Sure enough, my sex hormones were at rock bottom. They were lower than a postmenopausal woman, but I hadn't gone a year without my period. This was my wake-up call. I realized that the hormone hierarchy was real. If I didn't start working on cortisol production, I was never going to stabilize all the other hormones. I drew a line in the sand and decided self-care was going to become a top priority for me.

The steps I took to undo my rushing woman's lifestyle were so impactful for me that I now recommend these same steps to the women I coach one on one. If you know you need to stop the rushing woman's life you have created, I recommend you follow these steps as well.

Schedule Downtime

The first step I took in retiring the rushing woman was to build downtime into my schedule. But my schedule was jam-packed with work and family activities, so I looked for times that could accommodate more spontaneous unscheduled time. The beginning and end of the weekend held possibilities to slow down. I started with Friday and Sunday afternoons. Nothing got scheduled then. If I was invited to a social event during those times, the answer would be no. That was me time. Time for me to do whatever my heart desired. Sometimes that would be binge-watching a Netflix series; other times, I would go hiking with my husband. I gave myself permission to do whatever I wanted during these times without guilt or putting anyone else's needs ahead of mine. I started to crave this time. I found I had so much more joy the rest of my week knowing that downtime was already scheduled in. If you haven't done this for yourself, I highly recommend it.

Prioritize Self-Care

The second step I took to stop the rushing was to identify those activities that I loved doing and made me feel better, but often got pushed to the side because something more important got in the way. I needed to make those activities a top priority again. Two guilty pleasures I had were massages and facials. I often had an excuse as to why my schedule was too packed to fit them in. Once I made a decision to make myself a priority, I dropped those excuses. I immediately put a monthly facial and massage on my calendar. I told myself to look at those appointments as the most important appointments I had all month. Nothing more important would get in their way. I made a promise to myself that I wouldn't cancel them.

With these two steps firmly in place, I could feel my joy coming back. I slept better, relaxed easier, and enjoyed the times I rushed a whole lot more.

Adapt Your Workout Schedule

The third thing I needed to address in my rushing woman's life was my workout schedule. In my younger years, I was a competitive athlete. I have trained my brain to push on through any aches or pains I might experience in a workout. I also have learned how to override that voice that says, "Don't work out today; your body's not up to it." I decided to tune in to my body more and listen to what kind of workout it might need. Some days, I felt like going on a long run. Other days, I wanted to just take a walk in the sun. I started doing less push-on-through workouts and nurtured myself more with exercise like yoga and Pilates.

Practice Vacation

Don't get me wrong, I am still a rushing woman in recovery. Although I have made great strides to slow down, I still have more to implement. Last year, I told a good friend of mine who is a life coach that I would add to the previous steps by going on vacation more. One of my biggest challenges in slowing the rushing woman is that I love my life. I know that doesn't sound like a challenge, but when you say yes to all the exciting experiences that come your way, before too long, you're just rushing from experience to experience, never taking the time to enjoy each one.

Taking more vacations was a hard one for me. I know that sounds strange, but I have a lot of responsibilities. The thought of taking time off was paralyzing. Where would I fit it in? How will my patients do if I am not there for them? Won't the work pile up? I'll just have to come back to a long list of "have-tos." My friend had a brilliant recommendation for me. "Just practice vacation," she said. "Put it in your schedule, and if you're not ready at the scheduled time, move it to a different day. You're just getting used to vacation being on your schedule. Start there." That's what I did. Although I still can do better in this department, last summer I spent three weeks in Europe with family and friends. I've been in private practice for over 23 years and that's the longest vacation I have taken yet. Progress over perfection, right?

Get a Daily Dose of Oxytocin

With all the aforementioned changes in place, I still knew I had more to do to keep cortisol from taking over my body. I went back to the hormonal hierarchy. Oxytocin influences cortisol. What did I do to get a daily dose of oxytocin? This sent me down a path of research. What activities would I implement to get my body to secrete more oxytocin? It turns out this is a fun hormone to try to get more of.

Some of my favorite ways to secrete oxytocin are:

- Hugs
- Laughter
- Hanging out with friends
- Petting an animal
- Random acts of kindness

- Giving someone a gift
- Yoga
- Meditation
- Deep breathing
- Massage
- Chiropractic adjustment
- Listening to music
- Sex
- Connecting with others on social media

It's easy to look at that list and discredit how powerful each one of these activities can be for your hormones. I know I did before I understood how the hormonal hierarchy worked. But the more I prioritized oxytocin, the better I felt. One way I have used oxytocin in my favor has been to help me sleep. I find that something as simple as petting my dogs for a few minutes can bring my daily cortisol levels down enough to allow my body to fall into a deep sleep. I've also found that searching for moments where I can give a random act of kindness to someone has had a profound effect on my hormones. Now that I understand the massive importance of oxytocin, it's fun to give someone a hug instead of a handshake or to prioritize time to sit and laugh with friends. And these activities are not hard to do. You just have to remind yourself: oxytocin over cortisol. Fun over stress, all for the benefit of your hormones.

Show Your Adrenals Some Love

The last piece of understanding of how the rushing woman's syndrome was affecting my menopause journey came to me while sitting at a functional endocrinology seminar. The presenter pointed out that when the ovaries begin to shut down during menopause, they hand the job of making sex hormones over to the adrenal glands. If the adrenals are worn down from a rushing woman's lifestyle, they will be left depleted of progesterone and testosterone. This will leave the woman feeling tired and anxious, missing libido, and lacking motivation to workout. The presenter described my menopause journey to a tee. He then went on to explain how the precursor to cortisol, progesterone, and testosterone was DHEA. To bring your testosterone levels back up, you need to replenish your DHEA stores.

This was the final piece of my hormone puzzle. I couldn't understand where along my menopausal journey my testosterone had gotten so low. I went home that night and immediately revisited my DUTCH test. Sure enough, my DHEA levels were extremely low. I started on DHEA supplements right away, and within weeks I could feel my testosterone levels coming back up.

I share this story with you because I know many of you live this rushing woman's life as well. I see it in my patients and my online community. You try so hard to lose weight, get better sleep, and improve your moods. Yet you still feel stuck. If this is you, it's time to stop rushing. From one rushing woman to another, you've got this. Even if you feel like you can't slow down the responsibilities of your life, follow the steps I've laid out at the end of this chapter. As you loosen up your schedule and create more self-care moments, you will see how your menopause symptoms change.

The best place to start to unwind your rushed life is to work on these steps. Block out downtime on your schedule and guard it like it's life or death. Bring back those activities like pedicures and massages that may have fallen off your calendar. Put more vacations on your calendar. Find reasons to get more oxytocin surges throughout your day. Finally, if you haven't loved on your adrenals in a while, now is a good time. Something as easy as supplementing with DHEA can help you do that.

KATIE'S STORY

Katie came to me when she was in her late 50s. I often see postmenopausal women whose symptoms persist. At 57, Katie had increasing brain fog and fatigue, and her blood sugar was so unstable she found herself sleepy and crashing every afternoon. She thought she was living a healthy lifestyle, yet something was missing. Some part of her lifestyle was holding her back from being her best. We sat down together for a health consultation, and Katie pointed out that she was ready to take a leap forward in her health journey. She wanted to move her healing to a new level of prevention and longevity.

I first introduced Katie to a ketobiotic lifestyle with intermittent fasting. Immediately she felt a huge shift in her mental clarity. Her body streamlined, and she had energy like never before. Blood glucose levels also became easily manageable.

One benefit Katie discovered with this new way of eating was less anxiety. When she was in ketosis, she felt a calmness come over her. Katie had been an elite competitive figure skater in her younger years and no doubt was a recovering rushing woman. Her whole life had been about high performance. She had spent years learning tools to reduce her stress loads. Her current career is that of a high-performance coach, working with CEOs and elite athletes. She knew the importance of slowing the rushing woman down but adding keto-biotic to a less-stressed life took her recovery to a new level. This shift into more calm was a welcome change.

I watch so many rushing women struggle to bring their blood sugar down, even with the ketobiotic and fasting tools I teach. Cortisol has a powerful influence over insulin. What I learned in coaching Katie was that when you have an amazing toolbox for stress management and you add that to a ketobiotic fasting lifestyle, you will thrive. I have never seen someone get such quick results with the five steps of the Menopause Reset as Katie has. A large part of that is because of her mindset.

With a good foundation of ketobiotic, fasting, and mindfulness, I then introduced Katie to cycling in hormone-building days. Even though she was post-menopausal, she still needed to eat to build some estrogen and progesterone.

She loved the flexibility the hormone-building days gave her. She loved being able to get the benefits of ketosis while enjoying days filled with citrus fruit, sweet potatoes, and beans. This healing journey has been truly incredible for Katie.

At this point in her life, a few years post menopause, her body is doing better than ever. She is now ready to go to the next layer of healing, so I have been working with her to create a plan for treating her osteoporosis. She is the first to jump on all the biohacking equipment in my office. Her new treatment protocols include more detoxing, hyperbaric oxygen chambers, infrared sauna, red light therapy, and PEMF. Katie turns 60 this year, and with all the changes she made in her late 50s, she'll arrive at 60 more vibrant and healthier than ever before.

Steps to Slow Down the Rushing Woman

- Schedule downtime.
- Prioritize self-care.
- Adapt your workout schedule.
- Practice vacation.
- Get a daily dose of oxytocin.
- Show your adrenals some love.

You may wonder why I put this as the last step to your Menopause Reset. There is a specific reason for that. For many of the women I work with, this can be the hardest step. I want you to gain momentum with your health. If you start by changing what you eat and when you eat, you will feel immediate changes. Then move into feeding your microbiome and detoxing. Even more changes will come. If you finish your lifestyle makeover with resetting the rushing woman, your health will click into place and all the hard work you put into the first steps will elevate you to a whole new level. Just scheduling downtime won't have the same impact on your hormones if you don't follow the first steps. It's the synergy of the steps that will create magic in your life. I'm super excited for you. Please, reach out and find me on social media and share your results. Nothing excites me more than a menopausal woman who has gotten her life back.

Now that you have a foundation in lifestyle changes that will make a massive impact, I can't wait to share with you some new tools I've discovered that will keep you forever young.

CHAPTER 11

•••••••••••••••••••

Stay Forever Young

Everything I have taught you up to this point is what I consider lifestyle hacking. If you want to thrive throughout your menopause journey, applying these principles will help you take your health to a level you may never have known you were capable of achieving.

Now I want to introduce you to a term that is getting a lot of attention in the antiaging world. It's called *biohacking*. Biohacks have three common traits. They are shortcuts to a desired result, they are natural, and they work with your body's own intelligence. The world of biohacking is incredibly fascinating. There are so many new biohacking tools emerging every day it's hard to keep up with the research on them all. Perhaps what is the most exciting is the more these biohacks are made available to the public, the less dependent we become on drugs and surgery. This is so encouraging!

We live in an interesting time. There is more of a desire to slow down the aging process than ever before. Baby Boomers refuse to age as their parents did. Gen Xers watch seniors deal with dementia, Alzheimer's, and chronic arthritis at earlier ages and say, "Not for me."

People want to age differently. In this new world of bio-hacking, there are some exciting technologies (with a tremendous amount of research behind them) that can help the average person slow down the aging process. As you go through your menopause years, some of these tools may be of use to you. My favorites for the menopausal woman are red light therapy, infrared saunas, hyperbaric oxygen chambers, PEMF, vibration therapy, and brain training.

Before I map out each one of these exciting tools, a word of caution: your lifestyle will make or break you. Biohacking is not a replacement for a lifestyle that prioritizes the hormonal hierarchy. As tempting as it might be to jump into a hyperbaric oxygen chamber to solve your mood and memory problems, you will still need to address daily habits. It's the synergy of the biohack tools together with the lifestyle hacks that will have you thriving through your menopause years.

That being said, let me introduce you to some amazing biohacks that will slow down the aging process and help out your hormones.

Red Light Therapy

When you are inside all day sitting in front of your computer with fluorescent lights shining down on you, you are getting a large dose of blue light. Certain blue lights can be damaging to your cells and force them to age much quicker. This is especially true in the tissues that get exposed to blue light the most, like your skin. Yikes.

Not all light is damaging, though. There are healing lights that can invigorate your cells and help them live longer. Red light is one of those lights. You can naturally get red light when the sun rises and sets. But if you are like most people, you're not rushing outside to get this light on a regular basis. This is where red light therapy comes in handy.

Shining red lights on different parts of your body for as little as 10 minutes a day can have a profound effect on your collagen production and hormonal system and may even lower your joint inflammation. There are lots of great red lights out there; the one we use in our office is made by Joovv.

The research on this healing red light is profound. For menopausal women, collagen skin rejuvenation may be the most exciting result. Numerous studies show that red light therapy counteracts signs of aging in skin. Both red and near-infrared light have been shown to boost collagen, smooth wrinkles, and enhance skin tone, for an overall younger look.[11]

Red light therapy is also proving to have an effect on our endocrine glands (specifically, the thyroid). A three-year, randomized study done on 43 patients in Brazil proved that participants in the study who received red light therapy needed less thyroid medication than they normally needed. Many saw a decline in their thyroid antibodies.[12]

Infrared Saunas

Infrared saunas are an incredible tool for detoxification, weight loss, and skin rejuvenation. As you move through menopause, your toxic load may reveal itself. This can cause you to gain weight quicker than ever. Infrared saunas are a great tool to remove those toxins naturally.

Think of infrared light like a fever. It heats the cells up from the inside out. This heat encourages the cells to release the toxins they may be holding. Remember those receptor sites that get blocked with toxins? Infrared saunas can be a tool to unblock those receptor sites and get your hormones working again.

Infrared saunas are also used to repair aging skin. A study published in *The Journal of Cosmetic and Laser Therapy* showed significant improvements in skin appearance after just 12 weeks of sauna skin therapy using near-infrared technology. Participants experienced a reduction in wrinkles and crow's feet, as well as improved overall skin tone, including softness, smoothness, elasticity, clarity, and firmness.[13]

Lastly, we use infrared saunas a lot in our clinic for anyone going through our heavy metal detox programs. According to detox expert Dr. Dietrich Klinghardt, infrared mobilizes mercury in deeper tissues, making it an effective solution for removing mercury from the skin. Far infrared saunas are believed to be more effective in moving toxins through the skin than traditional saunas because in a far infrared sauna only 80 to 85 percent of the sweat is water with the non-water portion being cholesterol, fat-soluble toxins, toxic heavy metals, sulfuric acid, sodium, ammonia, and uric acid.[14]

Hyperbaric Oxygen Chamber (HBOT)

I call this my Benjamin Button machine. Remember that movie? Brad Pitt plays a character who ages in reverse. That's how I feel when I jump into the oxygen chamber in my clinic on a regular basis.

As you age, your cells become saturated with oxygen. It becomes difficult for you to drive more oxygen in, even with workouts like high-intensity training. But we need oxygen. It's healing to the mitochondria in our cells that produce ATP to give us energy. The only way you can drive oxygen into these aging cells is to compress it. Kind of like putting carbonation in a bottle. That's what an oxygen chamber is all about. It's compressed oxygen that can get into your cells to create a healing effect.

Although hyperbaric oxygen is often used for muscle recovery and athletic performance, we are seeing dramatic changes in brain health using hyperbaric oxygen. Your brain requires more oxygen than any other body part. When you put someone in an oxygen chamber who has had repetitive brain traumas or age-related memory loss, it's miraculous. The brain heals with oxygen.

The research on hyperbaric therapy is impressive as well. Hyperbaric oxygen treatments have been proven to stimulate angiogenesis, growing new blood vessels into tissue, and have been demonstrated to cause stem cell release from our bone marrow into our circulatory system.[15] Hyperbaric oxygen chambers have also been shown to suppress inflammation.[16] The chambers we use in our office are made by HBOT.

PEMF

You know how your cell phone loses its charge and needs to be recharged? Well, new research is proving that the same thing happens to the cells in our body. Only it doesn't happen over a few days; it happens over years. We call it aging, or we feel like we are just slowing down, but the truth is that the cells in your body are meant to keep you thriving to well over 100. They are not meant to slow down at 50.

There are many requirements of your cells, and one of them is electromagnetic energy. We get electromagnetic energy from the earth. Have you ever noticed that you feel more calm and peaceful after spending time in nature? That's because you got a good dose of the earth's electromagnetic energy, and it powered up your cells.

In today's world, our cells are attacked by toxins, poor nutrition, inflammatory fats, blue lights from our cell phones, and bad EMFs from Wi-Fi surging through our homes and offices. These damage our cells and cause them to lose power.

This is where pulsed electro-magnetic frequencies (or PEMF) come in. I like to think of PEMF as the equivalent to my phone charger, only for my body. When you sit in a PEMF chair, you are recharging your cells. This extra power is proving to help give the body the energy it needs to recover from chronic pain, chronic fatigue, and even depression.

According to research from Yale Medical University from as far back as 1932, the depletion of electrical energy from the body is the root cause of poor health. PEMF provides that missing energy to help the body regenerate naturally. If that's not exciting enough, the FDA has also approved PEMF devices for bone growth. This is helpful for the menopausal woman who is dealing with osteoporosis or healing a fracture.[17]

There are many PEMF products out there. The one we use in our office is a professional-grade unit called a PULSE bed.

Vibration Therapy

Have you noticed how you have to fight to keep muscle as you age? Well, let me introduce you to vibration therapy. It's an incredible tool for a woman moving through menopause. Vibration therapy has been around for some time, and you probably have a vibration plate at your gym but didn't realize it.

There are two reasons I love vibration therapy. First, when you stand on a vibration plate, you have to use hundreds of more muscles than you use just standing on steady ground. This is why fitness trainers love it. If you do a squat on a vibration plate, you force more muscles to work with less effort on your part. We use vibration plates in my office all the time to train people's postural muscles so they don't get that rounded, forward-head posture that comes with aging or chronic use of cell phones.

The second reason I love this therapy is because it forces your bones to be stronger. Vibration therapy encourages your bones to hold on to calcium and phosphorus. This can improve your overall bone density profile. Whole-body vibration has also been proven to increase the level of growth hormone and testosterone in the serum of postmenopausal women, preventing sarcopenia and osteoporosis.[18]

Brain Training

I saved two of my favorite biohacking tools for last. Remember how the rushing woman's brain is operating from a fight-or-flight state? I noticed in my clinic that sometimes a patient is stuck in fight- or-flight mode and can't get her brain out of the stress loop. This is exactly where biohacking comes into play.

When your brain is stuck in a constant stress mode, it is operating from an area of your midbrain called the amygdala. The job of the amygdala is to keep you safe and always be on the lookout for a crisis. When you are locked into this part of the brain, all it takes is a little stressor in your life for you to have a huge stress response. Too many people operate from this part of the brain all the time.

A better part of your brain to operate from is your prefrontal cortex. This is the part of the brain that can help you see hope and possibility. When you operate from your prefrontal cortex, you can set a goal and understand the steps and time it will take to achieve that goal. It is the center of your executive functioning.

Here's where things get really interesting: you can't think from both the amygdala and prefrontal cortex at the same time. Your brain is either operating from hope or fear. You get to choose from where you want to operate. The hard part is that if you have had a lot of trauma in your life or have been living a stress-filled life, you may be stuck in fear.

My two favorite brain biohacks can help get you unstuck. The first one is a chiropractic adjustment. Chiropractic has been around for over 100 years. It is not a new approach, but our understanding of how it changes the brain is new. Chiropractic was originally discovered by Dr. D. D. Palmer, a biomagnetic healer who understood how energy moved through the body. Dr. Palmer was one of the first to teach that the root of all disease was a decrease in nervous flow due to the presence of traumas, negative thoughts, and toxins. The more physical, emotional, and chemical stress you have, the more ill your body would be. He was the first to discover that when you adjusted the spine, you activated the nervous system and created a healing response in the body. For years, people have been going to chiropractors to speed up healing and prevent disease.

In recent years, a researcher named Dr. Heidi Havvik discovered that one chiropractic adjustment can immediately pull the brain out of fight-or-flight mode and move activity to the prefrontal cortex. Her research proved that you get 30 percent more blood flow into your prefrontal cortex after a chiropractic adjustment.[19] This is incredibly helpful for the menopausal woman who is stuck in fight-or-flight.

The second biohacking tool we use in our office to retrain the brain is called BrainTap®. This is a technology created by Dr. Patrick Porter, author of *Awaken the Genius*. His BrainTap headset uses four key elements to induce brain entrainment. These elements include binaural beats, guided visualization, ten-cycle holographic music, and isochronic tones. All these elements have a tremendous amount of science backing their effectiveness. My patients like to call this biohack "forced meditation." It takes years to train your brain to work in a more balanced way. Because BrainTap exercises the parts of your brain that you don't use when you are stuck in fight-or-flight, it can change your reactions to stress in a matter of weeks.

I brought this tool into my clinic because I wanted to help give my patients another way to handle their stressful lives. The results they have been getting with BrainTap have blown me away. Kids are focusing better at school, stressed-out moms are noticing they don't react to stressors as quickly, and patients who have struggled with insomnia are finally falling asleep easily. It has been an incredible addition to our biohacking center. Many of our patients love BrainTap so much they get a headset for home use.

I have been so impressed with how the above biohacks speed up the healing process and help the menopausal woman that I built a whole clinic around these tools. We call it the Reset Room. It has become a place where people come to power up their body and reset the stressors life is throwing at them. The results people are getting with our Reset Room tools have truly been incredible to witness.

Steps for Staying Forever Young

- Put lifestyle hacks from the previous chapters in place first.
- Identify which biohacks you need.
- Go see a chiropractor.
- Find a biohacking center near you or buy equipment for home use.

For the first time in human history, people are refusing to age. A large part of this antiaging movement is coming from the Baby Boomer generation. They don't want to age as their parents did. They are awakening to the idea of preventive medicine. One of the major health conditions they want to prevent is aging. This has forced research and created a demand for new technologies that have now become known as biohacking. It's such an exciting time to be involved in the biohacking movement. The miracles we see in our office alone with red light, oxygen chambers, and PEMF are mind-blowing. If you think you have to age as your parents did, think again. The principles I taught you in this book, mixed with the results that many of these biohacks can give you, will no doubt keep you forever young.

CHAPTER 12

Move from Surviving to Thriving

At this point, you most likely fall into one of two different camps. The first camp is for the overwhelmed. If you don't know where to start, I get it. Hang in there. This chapter holds some solid steps to getting started and building a lifestyle that works for you. Alternatively, you might fall into the second camp: you've been doing a lot of what I mapped out here but discovered a few more pieces you can put into place. If this is you, I encourage you to stretch yourself and see what you can do to take your health to a new level.

Look at your health as a puzzle. Everyone's puzzle size is different. Some of you may only have a 250-piece puzzle to solve, whereas others may have a 1,000-piece puzzle. Either way, I want you to be patient. Just like when you tackle a big puzzle, you can start by pulling out the border pieces, then sorting by color, then building the border, and finally diving into the center of the puzzle. That's the same approach I want you to take with your health.

Let's start with the border pieces. Go back and review the chapters. What did you feel like you needed to do the most work on? Start with that chapter and that lifestyle change first. Go to the bottom of the chapter and work the steps.

A good friend of mine, Amy, was postmenopausal and wanted to try incorporating fasting into her health regimen. She'd had an eating disorder as a young child and was nervous about what fasting might do for her mindset. Yet she wanted to give fasting a try. I had her work the steps I teach in the fasting chapter. She started with the first step: push breakfast back an hour. Once she got comfortable with that, she tried going 13 hours every day with no food. Going 13 hours was tough, so she focused on that step until it felt easier. Within a month she got the hang of it and was ready to fast longer. Before she knew it, she was easily doing the dinner-to-dinner fast and loving it. If you are new to fasting, follow the steps that Amy did above.

Once you have mastered the steps of the first chapter you've chosen to work on, move to another chapter and work those steps in order. This is exactly what Amy did. She became such a fasting fan she wanted to know more. She felt so good she wanted that next level. The next level for her was to work the steps in Chapter 7. Being a sugar addict, she knew this next lifestyle change was going to be tough. But she followed the path I laid out for her: She removed refined carbohydrates first. Then she started counting macros for carbohydrates and protein. Then she cleaned up the quality of the food she was eating and added in more good fat. Each step took time to adapt and adjust to. Each step provided a new challenge but also a new level of health. Each step motivated her to do more. With her fasting lifestyle firmly in place and her carbohydrate load down, she was at her ideal weight, energized, and ready to start detoxing. This is the perfect approach to the lifestyle recommendations I make in this book. Step by step—by the time you know it, you love the body you are living in.

I realize that you may be an overachiever and want to take on more than one lifestyle change. I get you. That works, too. You can easily combine the steps of two or three chapters. This is what I do when I am working one on one with a patient. We look at how many changes they want to make, what their goals are, and what the demands of their life may be so we can create steps that set them up for success.

One lesson that social media has taught me is that the principles I teach here are so refreshing and effective that you are going to want to know as much as possible about how to apply them to your life. This means you most likely will have questions as you move through the steps. My YouTube, Instagram, and Facebook pages get thousands of questions from the community every week.

I wrote this book to save lives. The five-step process to the Menopause Reset will move you from a path of building disease to a path of building health. If the self-guided, stepped approach doesn't work for you, I do have resources you can tap into to make your journey a little easier. I have an online community of people who are all working these principles. Feel free to join me in any of these programs. There are three online programs available: the Resetter Collaborative, the Reset Academy, and the group detoxes. The Resetter Collaborative is my Facebook group that fasts together once a month; the Reset Academy is my online membership group where I teach fasting variations, diet variations, and microbiome repair; and my group detox program is where I guide you through a detox that will pull neurotoxins and carcinogens from your body. Pick which one feels right to you.

LISA'S STORY

• •

At 45 years old, Lisa's health was in a downward spiral. She was exhausted all the time, not sleeping, losing her memory, and filled with anxiety. Nothing could relax her. Even the smallest of stressors would send her into a panic attack. She had amazing kids, a loving husband, and a life that she loved. Her anxiety made no sense to her. Lisa knew she had to do something different, so she reached out to me for help.

I customized the Menopause Reset process. I spent several months working with her to build the right fasting lifestyle that fit into her schedule. Her weekends were packed with her kids' sporting events, so fasting became a valuable tool for her on those long days. I taught her how to get into ketosis, which provided her with a tremendous amount of energy and mental clarity and helped her lose that last 20 pounds she had been trying to get rid of for years. She tested her toxic load and went through several customized detoxes with me, which made her feel calmer and put her sleep back on track. Within a year of our first meeting, Lisa was a more vibrant, calmer, and happier version of herself. She took the tools I taught her and built herself a lifestyle that had her thriving through menopause. Lisa is now 50 years old and told me the other day that she has officially gone a year without her period. As she sat in my office talking about how she felt to officially be postmenopausal, she reflected on her menopause journey. She said, "You know, going through menopause wasn't that bad for me." It was such a beautiful moment for both of us because Lisa realized that since she'd course-corrected her lifestyle at 45, she hadn't experienced the turbulence menopause can cause in so many women.

Steps to Putting It All Together

- Pick the lifestyle change you need to work on the most.
- Work the steps of that lifestyle change in the order I gave them.
- Once you've mastered one lifestyle change, move on to the next lifestyle chapter you are drawn to.
- Work the steps of that chapter, and so on.
- If you need more structure or community support, join the Resetter Collaborative and/or my Reset Academy.
- Get further tests or a health consultation to customize your approach.

If you still feel lost, please reach out. I have an amazing team of caring people who are here to support you and get you pointed in the right direction. It might be that you need to do more testing to understand your body better, or perhaps you need a one-on-one consult to help you figure out which pieces are missing in your health puzzle. No matter where you are on your health journey, know that you can heal.

As I moved through my 40s, so many of my imbalances showed up. It took me most of that decade to discover what I just mapped out for you in this book. Too many women struggle through menopause and are given few answers. You can fix many of your symptoms with lifestyle changes, but it doesn't have to take 10 years. I want you to feel better now.

Whether you work the steps in each chapter or join me in one of my programs, know that I am cheering you on.

Menopause is an incredible time to course-correct your life. Look at your symptoms as cries for help. When you understand how to address your symptoms with changes made to your lifestyle, the cries will stop. Most importantly, you will feel in control again.

CHAPTER 13

•••••••••••••••••••••

You Are More Powerful Than You've Been Taught

Whew! You have made it to the end. I hope the journey I have taken you on in this book excites you and gives you hope again. I wish you could stand where I am standing and see the thousands of success stories I've witnessed of women who reset their menopause symptoms following the five steps I laid out for you. Remember each chapter holds a different layer of healing for you.

If you find yourself lost on your menopause path, revisit Chapters 4 and 5, where I taught you about the hormonal hierarchy and which hormones are affecting your symptoms. If you are struggling with your weight, energy, hot flashes, or mental clarity, reread Chapters 6, 7, and 8 and start to create a fasting and ketobiotic lifestyle for yourself.

Tired of not sleeping? Losing your hair? Do you feel like your memory is not what it used to be? Then go back to Chapter 9 and familiarize yourself with the toxins in your environment that might be throwing your hormones off.

Lastly, if you can't seem to lower your blood sugar or you feel that you are doing everything possible to make your symptoms go away but nothing is working, reread Chapter 10. It might be time to slow the rushing woman down.

As you work this five-step process, never forget that the miraculous body you were born in comes preprogrammed to heal. Your body is way more powerful than you've been taught. I know the struggles you've been going through don't feel miraculous, but I promise you that in this wild menopause journey, there is an incredible opportunity to heal.

Menopause is a mirror. The symptoms that are staring you in the face are gifts that your body is asking you to address. My deepest hope for you is that you don't villainize these symptoms but embrace them. They are not happening to you, they are happening for you.

My heart aches for the health of our world today. But no one is more vulnerable than the woman moving through menopause. Hormones are protective. When you lose that protection and move into your postmenopausal years, you expose yourself to all kinds of diseases. Osteoporosis, hormonal cancers, cardiovascular disease, arthritis, dementia, Alzheimer's, and diabetes are all conditions that are more common in your postmenopausal years. As you sit in the transition from peri- to postmenopause, you have an opportunity. You can change the direction your health is heading. Implementing the lifestyle changes I laid out here can give you control. Chronic disease doesn't happen overnight. It takes years of a poor lifestyle for cancer cells to develop. When you tune in and listen to the needs of your body, disease stops building.

It doesn't matter what diagnosis you've been given, how many toxins you've been exposed to, or how many doctors gave you a poor prognosis, your body wants to heal. It's ready for this moment. It wants to work with you, not against you. There is powerful intelligence inside you that knows what to do. As you apply the five steps I mapped out in this book, you will see just how powerful your body was born to be.

You now have the tools to thrive throughout your menopause years. If you feel like you are getting off course, come back to the pages of this book. Revisit the chapters that explain your hormones. Remind yourself about the hormonal hierarchy and remember that when you balance cortisol and insulin, you will have more success balancing estrogen, progesterone, and testosterone. If you get lost and feel like your symptoms have a hold on you, come back to the five steps that make up the Menopause Reset. Look at these steps as a map for you to find your way out.

I see healing happen every day in my clinic. Women who have been stuck in their weight-loss efforts, are on multiple medications, or are losing their memory, struggling with sleepless nights, and chronically fatigued finally turn their health around. Not because of a magic pill or surgery. They turn their health around because they decided to believe in themselves again. They learn how to build a fasting lifestyle. They apply the principles of a ketogenic diet. They eat for their cycle when it shows up. They start caring for their estrobolome. They detox. They end the rushing. They commit to working with their body, not against it, and miracles happen. The body heals.

My favorite moment is when a patient says, "You know, this works." Yes, it works because your body was designed to work. You've just never been taught how to treat it.

Menopause is an opportunity to believe in yourself and make yourself the priority again. For many of you,

you have devoted the past few decades to your family, careers, or the needs of everyone around you. Now you get to devote this next phase of life to you.

Disease happens when we are disconnected from our bodies. This is easy to do. We live in a world that is more focused on external experiences. We ignore what is happening to us internally. We don't slow down enough to hear what our bodies are saying to us. Sometimes we just push on through our symptoms, never taking the time to listen. But when you stop to appreciate what is happening to your body throughout menopause, you'll be in awe. You have a major organ that has served you well for years that is slowing down. She's done her job. There is something symbolic and miraculous about that process.

I remember that one morning I sat in meditation after dealing with an especially tough few hormonal days. I was exhausted from the highs and lows of this journey. Frankly, I wasn't feeling enlightened that morning. I was angry at my body. I wanted my menopause madness to end. As I sat quietly, this thought came to me: "Don't be angry at your ovaries; they helped you make two beautiful children." It occurred to me at that moment that this incredible body part had a masterful hand in bringing me two of the greatest sources of joy in my life, my children. Every month, these ovaries showed up for me. They had a purpose that I greatly benefited from. Now it was time for them to retire. When I shifted my focus from anger to awe, all I could feel was a deep gratitude for these miraculous organs. I started to look at my menopause symptoms as a message from an old friend.

Our society has a clinical approach to this time of life. Symptoms are looked at as inconveniences that we need to make go away. If there is one thing my menopause journey has taught me, it's to honor these symptoms and the experience my body is going through. We are so blessed as women to live in a body that has had a hormonal symphony that has been going on month after month.

You can't heal a body you hate. As you move to the next phase of your life, make a decision to also move to gratitude and love. Honor the wisdom of this body you've been blessed to live in. When you come from a place of love and appreciation and combine that with building a lifestyle that works with you and not against you, you will thrive.

From the bottom of my heart, I hope this book helps. I believe in you. I know that the next phase of your life can be the best yet. Don't give up. I'm cheering you on.

●●●●●●●●·············

Effortless Sleep

If you had asked me in my 20s what my favorite pastime was, I would have told you sleep. Falling asleep, staying asleep, sleeping while traveling—you name it, sleep was an effortless health habit that I enjoyed thoroughly. When I hit my 30s, and I was learning how to balance motherhood and career, I discovered the power of the 20-minute nap. In those years, between the demands of my practice and nonstop duties as a parent, my days were in constant acceleration. A quick nap became my go-to antidote to my rushing woman's life. On a schedule-packed day, I learned I could rejuvenate myself with short bursts of sleep, so I built 20-minute naps into my lunch breaks where I quickly fell asleep and woke up rested and ready to go for the second half of my day.

Then my 40s hit and my relationship with sleep dramatically changed. The first huge shift I noticed was that I could no longer stay asleep all night long. Two in the morning became my witching hour. Instead of effortlessly falling back to sleep as I did in my younger years, I would toss and turn for hours while my brain hyper-focused on solving problems. In these early morning hours, my mind felt like a wild dog locking onto a bone. The obsessive looping of my thoughts would leave me awake for hours. Then I turned into this incredibly light sleeper. Noises from my family, my husband coming to bed late, and even the wind outside my window startled me out of my dreamy state. Trouble staying asleep eventually turned into trouble falling asleep. I could no longer put my head on the pillow and fall asleep easily. Instead, I would toss and turn for hours until my body and mind would let go and allow me to slip into a slumber. It was hell. Never in my wildest dreams did I imagine something I did effortlessly for years would become so difficult to achieve.

Just when I thought my sleep challenges couldn't get any worse, the night sweats kicked in. Trouble falling asleep, small noises waking me up, and nightly hot flashes left me an insomniac. I couldn't get a break. Figuring out how to get my hormone-depleted body to find its rhythm with a good night's sleep became my obsession. With the bliss of sleep turning into an arduous task, I set out to find new tools that would allow me to have a restful and restorative slumber. My frenzied sleep patterns launched me into a decade-long quest to discover what the menopausal body needs to be able to get a consistent night's sleep.

In this chapter, I want to share with you what I discovered. There are some game-changing sleep tools you need to know as you move into your menopausal years. Not only have these tools worked incredibly well for me but they have worked seamlessly for the thousands of women in my community. As I walk you through these tools, I want you to remember that insomnia is one of those conditions that seems to require a larger toolbox than other menopausal symptoms. One night you pull out one tool and it works like a charm, while another time it doesn't seem to have the same effect. That's okay. Don't give up on that tool. Unlike the other five lifestyle changes I've mapped out for you in this book, sleep tools are very dynamic. You won't be using all of them at the same time. Some nights you will pull one tool out, other nights you'll pull them all out. Sleep is one of those health habits you can't muscle your way through. Just as your hormones have a rhythmic flow to them, think of these tools as having a natural rhythm as well.

To help you better understand when to use these sleep tools, I have broken them down into three categories: foundational, strongly encouraged, and beautiful add-ons. Before I dive into these three categories in detail, I first want to walk through why menopause throws such a curveball in our sleep. Knowing why insomnia is showing up during your menopausal years will help you understand which of the sleep tools will work best for you.

Why Do Menopausal Women Struggle to Sleep?

Just like weight loss is hormonally dependent, so is sleep. There are five hormones that impact your sleep: cortisol, melatonin, insulin, estrogen, and progesterone.

Let's start with your sex hormones: estrogen and progesterone. It turns out these beautiful neurochemicals have been key in supporting you in a good night's sleep. As they start to decline, the simple act of falling and staying asleep dramatically shifts. One of the more spectacular qualities of progesterone is that she can activate GABA receptor sites in your brain, which allow your body and mind to relax. Without progesterone, your GABA levels can plummet, leaving you restless and struggling to sleep. The GABA and progesterone decline that accompanies menopause often feels like you've drunk several cups of coffee. You crawl into bed feeling tired, but once your head hits the pillow you feel wired and unable to relax. That is the loss of progesterone and GABA. When I go through the Beautiful Add-Ons section, I will give you many tools for raising GABA to allow you to effortlessly adapt to the low progesterone you experience after 40.

Estrogen loss is to blame for night sweats or hot flashes. During your menopausal years, estrogen dramatically swings, moving from moments where she is surging in at full force one day and plummeting the next. This estrogen roller-coaster ride is very common in the early part of your perimenopausal years. One day you will feel as if estrogen is your best friend giving you great mental clarity, the ability to multitask, laser-sharp cognition, smooth wrinkle-free skin, and full healthy hair. The next day you feel completely the opposite. Your mental focus is gone, skin and mucosal membranes dry out, and every stressor in your life seems to leave your brain in a state of fight-or-flight. It is these dramatic swings in estrogen that initiate hot flashes, especially at night. A sharp decline in estrogen signals your hypothalamus to turn up the heat. In one night alone, the highs and lows of estrogen can be extreme, leaving you drenched at multiple times throughout the night. If this is you, pay close attention to the foundational tools that I map out for you, because stabilizing estrogen's swings can be easily attained with some simple changes to your lifestyle.

Although melatonin is wildly known as the sleep hormone, getting your body to produce melatonin is not as easy as you would think. There are many aspects of your health that contribute to melatonin's production, but perhaps the most surprising trigger of melatonin release is your exposure to sunlight. Melatonin is light dependent. She makes her debut when your eyes register different types of light. Sunrise and sunset have more red light than other times of the day. These are the two times in the day that have the greatest influence on melatonin. In the morning as the sun is rising, the red hues that fill the sky tell your body to stop the production of melatonin. It takes a few hours in the morning for melatonin to slowly pause. At night when your eyes see the dusk sky darken, the red light that comes with sunset signals melatonin to rev back up because the day is ending and sleep is near. Midday light acts like a north star for melatonin, telling her where you are in your daily cycle. Resetting your circadian rhythm is pivotal for a good night's sleep. If you miss out on these three key light times, your melatonin levels may suffer. In the Foundational Sleep Tools section, I give you tried-and-true tips for resetting your circadian rhythm to allow your body to make melatonin, without leaning into supplementation.

Cortisol is the enemy of every aspect of your health, especially your sleep. Remember cortisol signals to your brain that there is a crisis at hand. And in a crisis, sleep is not in your body's best interest because survival is your body's top priority. When cortisol comes surging in, your body wants you to get up and go. It's time to run from that tiger. You may have experienced cortisol's need to flee during periods of chronic stress. When stress is consistently high, you can hit your pillow at the end of the day and find your heart racing and your body unable to let go enough to fall asleep. This happens because your hypervigilant body wants you to run, not sleep. If you wake up consistently at two in the morning, this also can be a cortisol surge knocking at your door. Usually, around two or three in the morning, your blood sugar is dipping toward its nighttime low. This dip in glucose can trigger hyperactive adrenals to give you a cortisol rush. This is no doubt the case when you wake up with your heart racing. This pattern of cortisol surging at the wrong moments of the day is called cortisol dysregulation. In both the Foundational Sleep Tools and Beautiful Add-Ons sections, I give you proven tools to balance cortisol so she doesn't activate your survival centers and wake you up.

The last hormone that affects your sleep is insulin. We often don't talk about high insulin causing a poor night's sleep, but insulin has an inverse relationship with melatonin. When melatonin is low, as during the day, you are more insulin sensitive. This means that anything you eat while it's daylight will have a better insulin response. This is important because insulin's job is to move glucose into your cells. The food you eat when it's dark out will not have the same insulin response, leaving extra glucose swimming in your bloodstream looking for a place to go. If you eat a high-carbohydrate meal at 8 P.M. in the wintertime, when it's dark out, the glucose from that meal will most likely move into fat stores and your brain tissue. Not only do large glucose spikes at night lead to more fat accumulation, but an increase in glucose can activate your fight-or-flight nervous system, telling your body it's time to be awake, not asleep. In the Foundational Sleep Tools section, I give you ideas on how to move your eating window around to time it to light exposure, not only allowing melatonin to rise but to give insulin the opportunity to regulate glucose more appropriately.

Foundational Sleep Tools

One of the most foundational sleep habits I had to face head-on in my 40s was resetting my circadian rhythm. As humans, our hormonal production is intimately tied to light production. This is the case for both men and women. But for the menopausal woman, it's even more important. As you lose the sex hormones that have helped you sleep, your body is forced to rely on other hormones and neurotransmitters to get the sleep job done. The neurochemicals in your body act like a team. If a couple of the members of the team are down, the others must step up and carry the extra load. This makes resetting your circadian rhythm vitally important during these years. When your body and mind are in circadian precision, your other hormones can properly flow in and out, giving your body the necessary neurochemical rhythm to get a good night's sleep.

Your Circadian Rhythm

Your circadian rhythm is the physical, mental, and behavioral changes that respond to the 24-hour-day schedule. It's your body's awareness of where you are in your sleep-wake cycle. This cycle is controlled by neurochemicals, both hormones and neurotransmitters, that are released throughout a 24-hour period to help you be alert during your day and sleepy at night. This system is hugely impacted by several outside influences, most importantly your exposure to light.

The best way to understand your circadian rhythm is to walk through what neurochemically happens to you in a 24-hour-day/night cycle. What I am hoping you will see as I map out a typical day is that there are a lot of outside daily influences that can throw off the neurochemicals that affect your sleep. Understanding this rhythm, and how to sync your daily habits with it, is critical for a good night's sleep.

When you first wake up in the morning, melatonin is still pulsing through your body. Your exposure to light turns melatonin off. Think of your exposure to light in the morning as turning on a circadian timer. Once the timer starts, your daytime neurochemicals begin to be released. Cortisol comes in first, slowly turning on the minute you get up, then hitting its daily peak two hours after you wake. Cortisol is a hormone that energizes you for your day. It also is a hormone that wants you to move. This makes the morning the best time to work out, from a hormone point of view. After cortisol peaks in the morning, it should naturally decline until it hits its daytime low in the early evening. If cortisol spikes happen in the afternoon due to stress, you can throw off this natural cortisol rhythm. This is called cortisol dysregulation and is a huge contributor to a poor night's sleep. One way you know you have cortisol dysregulation is that you feel wired and tired at the end of the day. Another common sign is a racing heart or strong heartbeat. If this happens to you at the end of the day, there is a good chance your cortisol pattern is dysregulated. It's hard to avoid stress these days, I get it. Often the stress keeps coming at us in the afternoon, causing cortisol spikes to occur when they shouldn't. Having said that, there are still some solid strategies you can insert into your stress-filled life that will help cortisol balance out so that you can sleep. Here are my five favorite ways to balance a rushing woman's cortisol levels.

Work with cortisol, not against it.

The first way to balance your cortisol pattern is to get up with the sunrise. The red hues of the morning sunrise shut off melatonin production. When you miss the opportunity for your eyes to see the red light in those early morning hours, melatonin will shut off abruptly upon waking and cortisol will spike quickly. For the menopausal brain that is adapting to the loss of hormones, a smooth gentle shift with your hormones is imperative. Abrupt changes in hormones can lead you directly into the hands of a poor night's sleep. Jolts to our hormones and nervous system take us out of our natural flow and put us in a constant state of fight-or-flight. Getting up with the sunrise and easing your way into the day balances both cortisol and your fight-or-flight nervous system to assist you in getting a good nighttime sleep. If you live somewhere that you can't see the red light of the morning, there are at-home red lights that you can turn on in the morning so your eyes will register the start of your day.

What you do in those early morning hours is important as well. If you go straight to your phone to check your e-mails, you are exposing yourself to blue light. Blue light will force melatonin to shut off abruptly. If your e-mails stress you out, cortisol gets activated. One simple act of getting on your phone first thing in the morning can throw off two major hormones. A huge daily habit I changed in my 40s was making sure I got up early enough to see the sunrise and then sit in my favorite chair to meditate and read something inspirational for the first hour of my day. I call this my miracle hour, as it worked miracles on both my mindset and sleep. Changing the way I start my day let me ease into it, aligning me with both melatonin's and cortisol's natural rhythms. This is such a powerful health habit that I still protect it carefully today.

Another critical step in letting cortisol naturally rise in the morning is the timing of your cup of coffee. Remember that two hours after you get up cortisol hits her peak. If you have a cup of coffee immediately upon waking, you will activate cortisol earlier than what is normal for your circadian rhythm. A simple step you can take to prevent this early production of cortisol is to wait two hours after you wake up to have your cup of coffee. Now, before you throw this book away after that comment, know that I get how crazy that sounds! I have been totally coffee addicted for most of my adult life. In my 40s, if you had told me to delay my coffee for two hours, I would have said that sounds like a torturous adventure I was not game for. Yet I found a simple strategy that eventually worked. I pushed my coffee back gradually each morning. Start by delaying it a half hour. Then a few days later push it back another half hour. Every few days move it back more and more. If you do that for several weeks, drinking your coffee two hours after you get up will feel more natural.

Another strategy I implemented in my 40s to balance my cortisol dysregulation was meditation. I moved straight from my bed to what I call my thinking chair to meditate. What I learned by delaying my coffee and meditating first was that my brain could get deeper into my meditation without the caffeine that my morning coffee provided me. Without caffeine, I could effortlessly tap into a brain-wave state known as theta waves. Theta waves are the brain waves that occur between the delta-wave states we experience with deep sleep and the beta waves we depend on to accomplish our daily activities. Theta waves are where inspiration and insight often kick in. It's a lot easier to meditate with your brain in a theta state. As I started to double-stack some of my circadian rhythm habits by delaying coffee and meditating first thing, my sleep dramatically improved.

Another cortisol regulation tool I adopted was moving my workout time to when cortisol was at its peak: two hours after I rose. Remember, cortisol wants you to move. This makes your morning workouts a powerful regulator of cortisol. Going for a walk or heading to the gym a couple of hours after you get up lets you use cortisol perfectly. Using cortisol when it comes flooding in is key for not only your sleep but overall health as well.

For afternoon spikes of cortisol that occur with stressful events, remember movement is a beautiful way to move cortisol through you. Get up and walk when a stressful situation occurs. This helps cortisol in two ways. First, you are putting this energizing hormone to its preferred use. Second, you are telling your brain that it doesn't need to stay in a fight-or-flight pattern. Anytime my mind moves into a place of fear or anxiety, I walk. I have found this to be one of the quickest ways to reduce anxiety and bring cortisol levels down.

Use the midday sun as a guiding light.

Once you have your morning routine synced to your hormonal needs, then you want to think of light exposure at other times of the day. Midday light, for example, tells your brain where you are in your day. If we go back to the idea that morning light starts the timer, then midday light tells your brain how many hours are left before sleep happens. If you are inside all day and don't get the full-spectrum light from midday, it can throw off your circadian timer. A quick 20-minute midday walk solves that problem. Midday light also activates serotonin receptor sites in your eyes. Serotonin is your feel-good hormone. It lifts your mood. Getting outside to let your brain register this full-spectrum light not only sets your circadian rhythm on the correct path but it brightens your mood as well.

As your afternoon continues, many of your energizing feel-good hormones start to decline. For example, cortisol hits new lows around 3 P.M. You may experience this as your afternoon crash. What's happening to you hormonally is that cortisol just plummeted. If you want a great night's sleep, resist reaching for a cup of coffee in the afternoon. This will no doubt put you on a path toward cortisol dysregulation.

Front-load your day.

What's interesting about the neurochemicals that are timed to our circadian cycle is that we have more energizing chemicals in the morning, while in the afternoon and evening these chemicals naturally disappear as our body prepares for sleep. Knowing this neurochemical rhythm, I have started to front-load my day. I get up at 5 A.M., do my miracle-hour morning routine, two hours into my morning I make a cup of coffee, then I move into my day. By 8 A.M. I am fully launched into work projects. After a few hours of work, I take a break to work out, but then jump right back into it. My goal is to be done with the most stressful part of my day by 4 P.M., which lines up with cortisol's natural rhythm. After 4 P.M., if possible, I move on to things that bring me joy and have an ease to them, like cooking, chatting with a loved one, or reading a new book. I realize you may not have a schedule that allows you to front-load your day, but if sleep is a serious struggle for you, see what you can do to front-load your higher-intensity activities. Front-loading your day's work will not only help you use the hormones that you need to conquer your day, but it will also protect you from the neurochemical imbalances that can often take place when the cortisol surges happen at the wrong time of day. Be playful with yourself as you implement this habit. Some days it may not be possible to block out stressful events. But if you are intentional about it, you will see that front-loading your day is fun, helps you focus on projects that need your concentrated energy, and gives you an opportunity to gradually ease into the hours before bed.

Dial in the proper evening light.

The last foundational idea I want to encourage you to implement is the routine you do in the hours leading up to bedtime. There are two major hormones to consider as you end your day: melatonin and insulin. At the end of the day, you want melatonin to be high and insulin to be low. That is how you were hormonally designed. When it's 8 P.M. at night, if melatonin is low and insulin is high, you will struggle to sleep. Let me give you some simple strategies you can implement to make sure that doesn't occur. First, be mindful of the light you are exposed to at the end of the day. Remember the red light in the sky at sunset signals to melatonin that it is her time to make her appearance. So if you have the opportunity to take a walk at sunset and watch the redness that fills the sky, that is an incredible melatonin boost. Second, once the sun has set, minimizing your exposure to blue light is key to a good night's sleep. Blue light turns off melatonin. Unfortunately, blue light is prevalent everywhere in your home. For starters, your LED lights that light up each room have waves of blue light in them. Your cell phone, computer screens, and TVs have blue light waves as well. So if you go for a walk at sunset hoping for a melatonin surge but come home to a house full of blue light, you might not feel the melatonin upswing your walk gave you. Luckily more of the world is catching on to the harmful effects of blue light and many gadgets have been made to block the blue light out at night. The easiest first step you can take is to get a filter to put your phone and computer screen into dark mode. Most phones and computers already come preprogrammed with light filters, but if yours doesn't have this feature, you can find downloadable filters that will block all blue light coming off your devices. The other trick that many use is to wear blue blocker glasses. This is a very easy step that allows you to block out all the blue light sources flooding your home at night. No matter which light-blocking path you take, know that your brain needs that shift in the spectrum of light it sees in the hours leading up to bed. Remember that a menopausal woman loses hormones that help her get a good night's sleep, so even though the blue light exposure in your home at night didn't affect your sleep in your 30s, it now may be impacting you.

Eat dinner earlier.

The timing of your dinner matters to your sleep. Insulin and melatonin work inversely. When melatonin goes up, you become more insulin resistant. When melatonin goes down, your insulin sensitivity is restored. What this means is that a dinner eaten too close to bedtime can shut off melatonin. A simple habit change of eating dinner earlier can keep melatonin working at her best. Many circadian rhythm experts strongly recommend that we should be consuming most of our food during daylight hours. This allows us to have better insulin sensitivity, creating a more balanced glucose response, plus it keeps melatonin shining at the right moments of your day.

Now, I realize that if you have never been taught about your circadian rhythm before, what I just mapped out for you may feel overwhelming. Hang with me here. There is an art to building a lifestyle around your circadian cycle. At the end of this chapter, I will give you steps to effortlessly incorporate the strategies I listed above.

Strongly Encouraged Sleep Tools

When it comes to sleep, it is common to desire a quick-fix tool. Yet quick fixes rarely give you lasting health results, especially when it comes to your circadian rhythm. There is a lifestyle that needs to be created in order to have consistent sleep night after night. That is why I mapped out the foundational tools first. Once you have your daily routine in sync with your circadian rhythm you are ready to add two other key sleeping tools that cater to your primal needs.

Your Primal Needs

Your body has a design that, when you work with it, will put you in the flow with health. Fasting and food variation, microbiome resetting, lowering your toxic loads, and calming your rushing woman lifestyle all have at their core a unique way of connecting you back to your primal design. Humans are at a moment in history where we are in an evolutionary mismatch with our modern world. Our constant access to food, overexposure to blue light, high-paced lives, and nonstop toxic influx have massively taken us off course with our health. This evolutionary mismatch is drastically hurting menopausal women. At a time when we are losing hormones, the stressors of our modern world are growing. A constant influx of physical, emotional, and chemical stressors pulls you away from your primal design and makes it hard for your menopausal body to rest at night. In this day and age, most women come roaring into their menopausal years already maxed out and living a stress-filled life. This modern, rushing lifestyle has a huge impact on sleep. To get your sleep back on track, you are going to want to mimic some of the habits of our primal ancestors. The light, food, and movement strategies I mentioned above begin that process.

Let's start by looking at what a cavewoman's sleeping habits might have been. For starters, women in the primal days had no choice but to be synced with the light rhythms of day and night. Yet there are two other huge sleeping steps these women took that we can learn from. They slept on the cold, hard ground with a heavy animal hide draped over them as a blanket. This is key because your body is designed to go to sleep when your core temperature drops, and your nervous system is built to calm down when a subtle weight is placed upon it. As crazy as it sounds, your body was designed to sleep well in the cold. This is especially key for the menopausal woman who has hot flashes all night long. Science is now proving to us that a signal to your brain that it's time to sleep is when your core temperature drops five degrees. There are several ways you can accomplish this.

First, you can turn up the air conditioner at night or open a window to let the cold night air into your room. This can be a fabulous relief for the menopausal woman who experiences hot flashes at night. If it's summertime or you live in a consistently warm environment without access to air-conditioning, I highly recommend something called a cooling mattress. This a mattress cover that cools down at night. In fact, you can set the temperature to the coldness you desire. As a menopausal woman, the most important part of regulating your temperature at night is that you make sure your body temperature stays on the cool side. I have been blown away by how some nights I crawl into bed after doing all the right sleep strategies, yet I still toss and turn. This is when temperature makes such a crucial difference. Often I just reach down to the controls on my cooling mattress, turn the temperature down a few degrees, and instantly fall asleep. It's quite miraculous for me. Now, if you don't like the cold, this may sound horrible. But I promise you that a small shift in your core body temperature is magic for your sleep.

The other sleep tool that mimics your primal ancestors' is a weighted blanket. When I first heard of a weighted blanket, it sounded horrible to me. I could not wrap my head around the idea that weight on top of me when I sleep would relax me. But when I dove into the research and put the info through my primal lens, I realized that extra weight might positively trigger a part of my primal design. Just like a small drop in core temperature activates sleep, it turns out that a small amount of weight on top of you does the same thing. Cold mattress, slightly heavy blanket . . . now you are sleeping like a cavewoman. I have found that the trick with weighted blankets is finding the weight that works best for you. When I first experimented with this sleep tool, it took me several tries before I found the right weighted blanket for me. The one that worked the best for me can be found on my website.

Beautiful Add-On

With your circadian rhythm back on track and your primal needs being met, you are now ready to explore some incredible supplements that can assist your sleep. Remember that a supplement is meant to be an add-on to a healthy lifestyle. It's common for us to reach for a supplement in hope that it will solve our immediate health problem. I can tell you with 100 percent certainty that there is no one-size-fits-all sleep supplement that will work for everyone. I also know that supplements work much better when the foundational steps are in place. When it comes to sleep I have found that the supplements that will assist you in sleeping through the night fall into two categories: nervous system relaxers and nutrient necessities.

Nervous System Relaxers

If you are in a state of fight-or-flight, you will not be able to sleep. It doesn't matter how many of the tools you use. Your body has no survival advantage to sleep if it thinks a tiger is chasing it. It will keep your sympathetic nervous system activated telling your brain it's time to get up and run. This is not the message you want your brain to get when you put your head on the pillow.

I was reminded of this in the first year of the pandemic. After a long stressful day at my clinic, I would come home and get into deep discussions with my husband about all the stressors that were going on in the world at that time. Many of these discussions left me agitated and angry. I started to notice that I couldn't get my mind to shut off when I crawled into bed. So I implemented a pact with my hubby that we had to table the stressful discussions after 8 P.M. I needed my nervous system to begin to wind down at this time. This one change to my nightly routine worked like a charm in letting me rest at night during a very stressful time.

Sometimes stressors keep coming at us. Our nervous systems never get a chance to kick out of fight-or-flight. This is when you need to reach for assistance. When it comes to soothing your frazzled nervous system, there are three supplement go-tos that I reach for.

The first go-to I recommend is a high-quality CBD supplement. Your body has an endocannabinoid system that balances both your nervous system and your immune system. If this system gets depleted, then your ability to switch out of fight-or-flight becomes near impossible. Since we live in a world where stress is high for so many, CBD supplements have become quite the rage. And with good reason! Adding a good CBD supplement a few hours before bed can really help you move out of a state of stress and into a more relaxed state.

How do you find the right CBD supplement for you? Finding the perfect CBD supplement is definitely a personal journey. That means you will need to experiment with what your body responds to best. A good general guideline to know is that you have several types of CBD receptors in your brain. Some respond best to straight CBD alone, other receptors are best stimulated with a small dose of THC mixed in. In recent years, the world of cannabis has gotten very sophisticated. Gone are the days of just taking straight CBD. For sleep and relaxation, I have noticed that my body does best with a mixture of CBD, CBN, and THC. But I only know this because I have spent years testing out which products work best for me. You can find my favorite CBD products on my website.

My second nighttime go-to is kava, a relaxing plant medicine. Used by islanders for centuries, kava can stimulate your parasympathetic nervous system. This is the part of your nervous system that calms you. So often we sleep poorly because we've underutilized that part of our nervous system. Just like a muscle that doesn't get used, if you don't train yourself to use your parasympathetic nervous system it will weaken. This makes it hard to switch gears on a day where you have been in a constant state of fight-or-flight. This is where kava can come to the rescue and be incredibly supportive to your parasympathetic nervous system. A cup of kava tea or a dropperful of a tincture turns on your rest-and-digest nervous system. It's a great tool to reach for after dinner. Turning on your parasympathetic nervous system at that moment of the day not only helps you digest your food but puts you in a more relaxed state.

The last nervous system relaxer I have found consistently helpful is a strange little fatty acid known as phosphorylated serine. This unique nutrient is known to lower your body's production of cortisol by 50 to 70 percent. I often use this nutrient at 2 A.M. when I wake up with my mind spinning. Taking a small dose at that moment lowers my cortisol levels, calms my anxious brain, and helps me fall back asleep. When my rushing woman lifestyle has soared to new heights, I make sure I always have this fatty acid with me. I've used it in the late afternoon when the stress of the day may still be in full force. I have taken it at 9 P.M. at night when I can't seem to relax enough to put myself in a sleepy state. For me, it feels like I activate a switch that immediately pulls me out of fight-or-flight and puts me right back in sync with sleep.

Nutrient Necessities

If all these sleep tricks aren't working for you, it may be time to look at possible nutrient deficiencies your body may have. The two most common deficiencies I have seen affect a menopausal woman's sleep are magnesium and melatonin.

Magnesium is a key mineral that you need to make many of your hormones, but most importantly progesterone. Of your sex hormones, progesterone is the one that helps you sleep. As you move through your menopausal years you lose progesterone, contributing to insomnia. The name of the menopausal game is to keep your age-appropriate sex hormones at their highest level possible. That means if you want to maximize progesterone's production, then it would behoove you to add magnesium.

There are many of different types of magnesium, as this powerful nutrient doesn't just support progesterone production but calms many of the tissues in your body. For example, magnesium citrate relaxes your intestinal tract, making it a great supplement for constipation. Magnesium threonate calms your brain during those anxious moments. When it comes to sleep, I recommend a supplement with a complete mix of different types of magnesium. You may have to try a few different types to dial in to the one that works for you. Because much of our food is grown in mineral-depleted soils, most of us are walking around with a magnesium deficiency. I can't tell you the number of menopausal women who found great sleep relief in taking a magnesium supplement right before bed. Try it for 30 days and see if you notice a difference. Many also report feeling like they get a deeper, more restful sleep on magnesium.

Ironically the sleep supplement I recommend as a last resort is melatonin. Let me tell you why. As powerful as melatonin is, you want to make sure your body is doing everything possible to make it on its own. If you add melatonin from an outside source, your body may slow down its own natural production. The name of the sleep game isn't to find the perfect supplement that you can never sleep without again. You want to do everything you can to get your body to naturally fall asleep and stay asleep. Once your body knows that there is an exogenous source of a hormone coming into your system, it can stop producing that hormone on its own. Many women experience this with thyroid medication. Once on a synthetic thyroid hormone, you have to stay on it as the natural production of that hormone slows down. This is why I recommend melatonin last. I want to make sure that we've exhausted all your body's own internal resources for making melatonin.

Having said that, if you have a true melatonin deficiency, taking a supplement will help you sleep while you identify the root cause of that deficiency. The best test for knowing if you have a deficiency is the DUTCH hormone test that I have mentioned several times throughout this book. There is no doubt it's my favorite hormone test for women. One reason is that it can tell you your melatonin levels. A melatonin supplement for deficient menopausal women can truly be the miracle cure for sleep.

Putting It All Together

Hopefully, you can see that I have mapped out an effortless sleep lifestyle here for you. When you hit menopause the sleep game changes. During this time, it's so common to get caught up in pill popping to ensure you sleep. I have had so many sleepless nights that I get the desire to find your perfect pill, whether through medication or supplementation. All you want is to just turn off your brain and relax your body at night. Seems like a simple desire. But for the menopausal woman, it's not that simple. There is a more complete picture of sleep that was necessary to give you. Hang in there. There are a lot of tools that I have outlined here. Be playful about experimenting with them. Find the tools that work best for you. If that tool stops working, don't give up on it, it may serve you later. Below I have listed out the steps I would encourage you to take to start to build an effortless sleep lifestyle that works for you. With time, experimentation, and a curious attitude, you will sleep soundly again, I promise!

Steps to Building an Effortless Sleep Lifestyle

- Wake up with the sunrise.

- Delay your coffee by two hours.

- Meditate first, check e-mail after.

- If possible, move your workouts to morning.

- Front-load your stressful activities to earlier in the day.

- Take a 20-minute walk to catch midday light.

- Take short 5-minute walks when stress hits in the afternoon.

- Eat dinner earlier to maximize insulin sensitivity.

- Be sure your eyes register the red hues of sunset.

- Wear blue blockers after dark.

- Get your body temperature to drop five degrees.

- Add in a weighted blanket.

- Find a CBD or kava supplement that works for you.

- Try phosphorylated serine at night to calm cortisol.

- Add a magnesium supplement.

- Test for melatonin deficiencies and add a supplement appropriately.

Endnotes

1. Ho, Kian Y. et al. "Fasting Enhances Growth Hormone Secretion and Amplifies the Complex Rhythms of Growth Hormone Secretion in Man." *The American Society for Clinical Investigation, Inc.* April 1988 vol 81, 968-975

2. Mihaylova, Maria M. et al. "Fasting Activates Fatty Acid Oxidation to Enhance Intestinal Stem Cell Function during Homeostasis and Aging." *Cell Stem Cell;* (2018) vol. 22,5: 769–778. e4.

3. Rangan, P. et al. (2019) "Fasting-Mimicking Diet Modulates Microbiota and Promotes Intestinal Regeneration to Reduce Inflammatory Bowel Disease Pathology. "*Cell Reports.* 3 March 2019. Vol 26, 10.

4. Adawi, Mohammad et al. "Ramadan Fasting Exerts Immunomodulatory Effects: Insights from a Systematic Review." *Frontiers in Immunology;* 27 November 2017 vol. 8: 1144.

5. Patterson, Ruth E. et al. "Intermittent Fasting and Human Metabolic Health." *Journal of the Academy of Nutrition and Dietetics;* (2015) vol. 115,8: 1203–12.

6. Bahijri, Suhard M. et al. "Effect of Ramadan Fasting in Saudi Arabia on Serum Bone Profile and Immunoglobulins." *Therapeutic Advances in Endocrinology and Metabolism;* (2015) vol. 6,5: 223–32.

7. Looker, Claire et al. "Influenza Vaccine Response in Adults Exposed to Perfluorooctanoate and Perfluorooctanesulfonate." *Toxicological Sciences: An Official Journal of the Society of Toxicology;* (2014) vol. 138,1: 76–88.

8. "Immunotoxicity Associated with Exposure to Perfluorooctanoic Acid (PFOA) or Perfluorooctane Sulfonate (PFOS)." *National Institute of Environmental Health Sciences, U.S. Department of Health and Human Services.* September 2016.

9. Desai, Maunil K., and Roberta Diaz Brinton. "Autoimmune Disease in Women: Endocrine Transition and Risk Across the Lifespan." *Frontiers in Endocrinology;* 29 April 2019 vol. 10, 265.

10. Darbre, Philippa D., "The history of endocrine-disrupting chemicals, Current Opinion in Endocrine and Metabolic Research, Volume 7," 2019

11. Wunsch, Alexander, and Karsten Matuschka. "A Controlled Trial to Determine the Efficacy of Red and Near-Infrared Light Treatment in Patient Satisfaction, Reduction of Fine Lines, Wrinkles, Skin Roughness, and Intradermal Collagen Density Increase." *Photomedicine and Laser Surgery;* (2014) vol. 32,2: 93–100.

12. Höfling, Danilo B. et al. "Low-Level Laser in the Treatment of Patients with Hypothyroidism Induced by Chronic Autoimmune Thyroiditis: A Randomized, Placebo-Controlled Clinical Trial." *Lasers in Medical Science;* (2013) vol. 28,3: 743–53.

13. B. A. Russell, N. Kellett & L. R. Reilly "A Study to Determine the Efficacy of Combination LED Light Therapy (633 nm and 830 nm) in Facial Skin Rejuvenation." *Journal of Cosmetic and Laser Therapy* (2005) vol. 7:3–4: 196–200.

14. Sircus, Mark Ac., OMD "Detoxification Through the Skin." *International Medical Veritas Association.* 6 March 2005.

15. Kawada, Shigeo et al. "Increased Oxygen Tension Attenuates Acute Ultraviolet-B-Induced Skin Angiogenesis and Wrinkle Formation." *American Journal of Physiology. Regulatory, Integrative and Comparative Physiology;* (2010) vol. 299,2: R694–701.

16. Novak, Sanja et al. "Anti-Inflammatory Effects of Hyperbaric Oxygenation During DSS-Induced Colitis in BALB/c Mice Include Changes in Gene Expression of HIF-1α, Proinflammatory Cytokines, and Antioxidative Enzymes." *Mediators of Inflammation;* (2016) vol. 2016: 7141430.

17. Ehnert, Sabrina et al. "Translational Insights into Extremely Low Frequency Pulsed Electromagnetic Fields (ELF-PEMFs) for Bone Regeneration After Trauma and Orthopedic Surgery." *Journal of Clinical Medicine;* 29 April 2019 vol. 8, no. 12: 2028.

18. Weber-Rajek, Magdalena et al. "Whole-Body Vibration Exercise in Postmenopausal Osteoporosis." *Przeglad menopauzalny = Menopause Review;* (2015) vol. 14,1: 41–7.

19. Lelic, Dina et al. "Manipulation of Dysfunctional Spinal Joints Affects Sensorimotor Integration in the Prefrontal Cortex: A Brain Source Localization Study." Neural Plasticity; (2016) vol. 2016: 3704964.

Index

Index

Index

Index

Acknowledgments

I remember one sleepless night in my early 40s, when I thought, "How do women handle years of this menopause craziness? There has to be a different way!" It was at 2 A.M. when I made a promise to myself to find that better way. Suffering through this experience was not what I was going to do. As soon as I made that decision, answers appeared.

Some of the most amazing people showed up in my life to guide me on my menopause path. The first was one of the greatest mentors of my career, Dr. Daniel Pompa. He taught me how to think. I know that sounds crazy, but for the past five years, I have been blessed to study health from this brilliant man. Dr. Pompa and I share a deep respect for the intelligence of the human body. His teachings have shown me that you always have to look beyond the symptom and go upstream to find the root cause of why the symptom occurred in the first place. I am so grateful for Dr. Pompa's unquenchable thirst to understand what prevents the body from healing and how we can tap into our body's own intelligence to speed up the healing process.

The second person who showed up for me on this journey was Andrea Siebert. Everyone needs a friend like Andrea in their life. When my menopause brain had me filled with anxiety and fear, Andrea was there to fill me with words of faith and trust. When I had moments where I struggled to put my own health puzzle together, Andrea was there to give me perspective and remind me of the healing power of self-love. I have no idea how I would have made it through menopause without her friendship and wisdom.

Then there is my sweet Jessica Siebenhaar. From the moment we first heard Dr. Pompa talk on the Cal Jam stage, Jessica and I knew our calling would be to detox the world. Jessica has an incredible superpower of turning my wild ideas into systems that help us best serve our community. Patients often ask me how I am able to accomplish so many things at one time, and the answer is Jessica. She has allowed me to stay in a visionary role at my office while she works out the details so we can put my vision into action. Along with saving the world together, traveling to some really random places to learn together, and working crazy long hours, we have had the craziest experiences together that have produced some of the best laughs of my life. There is no way I could help as many people as we do without her by my side.

I always tell people that if you have big dreams that you want to become a reality, you're going to need a mindset coach. For the past several years, Katie Peuvrelle has been that coach for me. Your mind can be your greatest asset or your worst enemy. Training that mind is key to keeping you on course. Some people have a personal trainer; I have a mindset trainer. Katie has helped me see the beliefs that were holding me back and given me a fresh way of thinking to be able to build the life I had only dreamed of. When I lacked clarity, Katie helped me see the next step to take so I could keep moving forward. I am so grateful for her wisdom and friendship.

I also want to give a shout-out to my team. I work with some of the most amazing, heart-based people who want to change the world. I love my peeps! Thank you, Dana, Cardinal, Eliza, Dr. Catie, Katelynn, Rachel, Debbie, and Pelin. I love serving health with you all!

Acknowledgments

I am so grateful to be married to my best friend, my hubby, Sequoia. He is my rock. I am a verbal processor, and no one has put up with my verbal processing more than Sequoia. He is patient, kind, and is always there to be my sounding board. When I have been at my lowest, he has picked me up and cheered me on. He has believed in me when I didn't believe in myself. I feel so grateful to have raised two children and run multiple businesses with this amazing man. I adore doing life with him!

Finally, I want to thank you, the reader. I wrote this book because many of you asked how to apply the principles I teach on social media to your menopause experience. Thank you for being brave enough to find another answer to your health. I hear from thousands of you every week, and so many of you are looking for answers to your symptoms that don't require medications. That gives you control back. You know that there is a wisdom inside you that wants to heal you. Yet, you are unsure how to tap into that wisdom. Instead of relying on a pill or surgery to fix you, you are asking yourself, "What can I do to help myself?" I applaud you! This is absolutely the right question to ask. This book is my gift to you. From the bottom of my heart, I truly hope this book gives you hope and helps you discover just how powerful your body is designed to be.

About the Author

Dr. Mindy H. Pelz, D.C., is a best-selling author, keynote speaker, and nutrition and functional health expert who has spent over two decades helping thousands of people successfully reclaim their health. She is a recognized leader in the alternative health field and a pioneer in the fasting movement, teaching the principles of a fasting lifestyle, diet variation, detox, hormones, and more. Her popular YouTube channel, where she regularly updates followers on the latest science-backed tools and techniques to help them reset their health, has had more than 24 million lifetime views. She is the host of one of the leading science podcasts, *The Resetter Podcast,* and the author of three best-selling books, *Fast Like a Girl, The Reset Factor,* and *The Reset Factor Kitchen.* Dr. Mindy has appeared on national shows like *Extra TV* and *The Doctors,* and has been featured in *Muscle & Fitness, Well + Good, SheKnows, Healthline,* and more.

To learn more about Dr. Mindy and her work, visit drmindypelz.com.

You can also follow her on several different social media platforms where she uploads new material every week:

YouTube Channel: youtube.com/drmindypelz

Facebook Page: facebook.com/drmindypelz/

Resetter Collaborative: facebook.com/groups/resetters/

Instagram: @dr.mindypelz

Hay House Titles of Related Interest

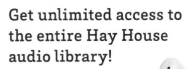
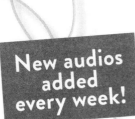

CONNECT WITH
HAY HOUSE
ONLINE

🌐 hayhouse.co.uk   f @hayhouse

📷 @hayhouseuk   🐦 @hayhouseuk

▶ @hayhouseuk   ♪ @hayhouseuk

Find out all about our latest books & card decks • Be the first
to know about exclusive discounts • Interact with our authors
in live broadcasts • Celebrate the cycle of the seasons with us
• Watch free videos from your favourite authors •
Connect with like-minded souls

'The gateways to wisdom and knowledge
are always open.'

Louise Hay